Table of Contents

The Immunity Code: Fuel Your Body Lifestyle ....

Dedication 2

Introduction 3

Nourishing Your Immune System with Real Food 6

Why Whole Foods Beet (okay, "Beat") Supplements 11

Hydration—A Key Player in Immune Health 19

The Critical Role of Sleep in Immune Health 25

Building the Foundations of Immune Health 31

Bringing Relaxation Practices into Your Daily Routine 34

Physical Activity and Immune Health: Move for Better Immunity ... 37

Advanced Strategies for Immune Support 40

Hygiene and Environmental Factors: Strengthening Immune Health Through Smart Habits 45

Habits vs. Willpower. Stress Reduction Habits for Better Health: Aka Your Brain and Behavior 50

Personalized Immune Support Plan 56

BONUS CHAPTER! | Childhood Health and Immune Wellness .. 59

Building a Foundation for Lifelong Health 66

Conclusion: A New Chapter in Your Health Journey 93

Appendix A: Nutritional Yeast 95

Appendix B: Resources and further reading:...98

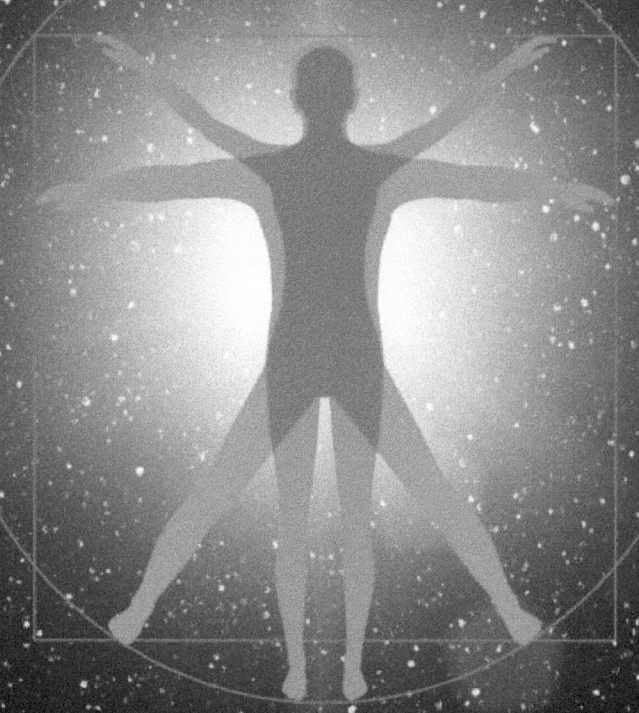

The Immunity Code
Fuel Your Body's Defenses with Food and Lifestyle

Michaela Gaffen Stone

Copyright © 2024 by Michaela Gaffen Stone

All rights reserved. No part of this book may be reproduced, distributed, or transmitted in any form or by any means, including photocopying, recording, or other electronic or mechanical methods, without the prior written permission of the publisher, except in the case of brief quotations embodied in critical reviews and certain other noncommercial uses permitted by copyright law. For permission requests, write to the publisher, addressed "Attention: Permissions Coordinator."

Published in the United States of America

Disclaimer

Before you implement or use any dietary, exercise, or health advice or suggestions from this book, please consult with a medical practitioner or qualified health professional.

You should not rely on any information provided herein as a substitute for, nor as a replacement for, professional medical or psychological advice, diagnosis, or treatment.

All information provided in this book is intended for educational purposes only. Any health or dietary advice is not intended as a medical diagnosis or treatment.

None of the statements made by the host or guest on the book have been reviewed or approved by the FDA.

The Immunity Code: Fuel Your Body's Defenses with Food and Lifestyle

Michaela Gaffen Stone

Dedication

This book would not have been written without the encouragement and editing/publishing help of my husband and best friend, Adam Gaffen. Thank you for prodding me (with both love and well-placed nudges) into turning all these thoughts into written words. Without you, this book would still just be a very long dinner conversation!

Introduction

In today's world, maintaining strong health is more important than ever, and our immune system plays a central role in defending against illness and keeping us vibrant. Yet, with the stress of modern living, and with food companies adding more and more chemicals into the products they sell, many of us are unknowingly weakening our immune defenses, making it crucial to take intentional steps to nurture and support our body's natural protection. There is a LOT to navigate!

I'm Michaela Gaffen Stone, the expert behind this guide, and I'm a seasoned nutrition coach and Board Certified Behavior Analyst with a passion for transforming lives through the power of nutrition and behavior change. With numerous certifications, including a Level 2 Master Nutrition Coach, I blend nutrition science with practical strategies for long-lasting health transformations. My unique perspective, at least partially shaped by my experience living in eight countries, allows me to offer a truly holistic and globally-informed approach to wellness. Now based in the U.S., I have helped countless individuals break free from unhealthy eating patterns, develop positive relationships with food, and embrace self-care that lasts a lifetime.

"The Immunity Code: Fuel Your Body's Defenses with Food and Lifestyle" is more than just a collection of facts and advice—it's an invitation to take control of your health and arm yourself with practical tools and insights. This book aims to demystify the inner workings of your immune system, showing you how to nourish your body from the inside out. With evidence-based guidance on essential nutrients like vitamins, minerals, antioxidants, and probiotics, I walk you through exactly what your body needs to stay strong and resilient in the face of illness.

But it doesn't stop there. This guide also focuses on the power of lifestyle changes—how simple habits like quality sleep, regular movement, and effective stress management can create a solid foundation for immune health. My comprehensive approach ensures that you're not just making changes in the short term, but building lasting habits that will support your immune system for years to come.

And because knowledge without action is only half the battle, I've included a delicious array of immune-boosting recipes, designed with both kids and adults in mind. These recipes make it easy—and enjoyable—to incorporate nutrient-dense, whole foods into your daily routine. From energizing breakfasts to comforting dinners, you'll have plenty of inspiration to fuel your family's health while indulging in flavors everyone will love.

This book is your go-to resource for understanding how the immune system works, how to nourish it with the right foods and habits, and how to lead a life that prioritizes wellness from the inside out. Whether you're looking to improve your family's overall health, or you're simply curious about how to make better choices to support your immune system, this guide will empower you with knowledge, confidence, and practical steps to take action.

Let's unlock the secrets to building a healthier, more resilient you—starting today!

Nourishing Your Immune System with Real Food

The immune system is one of the most complex and vital functions of the human body, tirelessly working to protect us from illness, infections, and disease. And while there's no shortage of products that claim to boost immunity, the real foundation of a healthy immune system begins with what we eat. Almost as important? What we *don't* eat. By focusing on nutrient-dense, whole foods, we can equip our bodies with the tools needed to fend off illness and keep us functioning at our best. In this chapter, we'll explore how vitamins and minerals play a crucial role in building and maintaining a strong immune system for everyone in your family. Young or old, we *all* need to eat right!

Getting real (not chemical) vitamins and minerals from real, unprocessed foods not only ensures that they're absorbed more efficiently but also provides additional health benefits that supplements simply can't offer.

Now, I don't plan to leave you with a vague idea of how to 'eat right'. For one thing, maximizing your immune health - cracking that code - is about much more than your food. We're going to explore exactly what the Immunity Code is all about and what it means for you - without breaking the bank. To begin, let's look at the key vitamins and minerals that support immune health, where to find them in your everyday diet, and why getting your nutrients from food is always the best choice.

Vitamin A: Your Body's First Line of Defense

Role in Immunity

VITAMIN A IS ESSENTIAL for maintaining the health of your skin and mucous membranes - for example those seemingly easily infected linings of your nose and throat - which act as barriers to infections. It also plays a vital role in developing and maintaining your immune system, particularly in the production of white blood cells. These are the body's frontline defenders, attacking and eliminating harmful invaders like bacteria and viruses.

Great Sources

TO ENSURE YOUR FAMILY gets enough Vitamin A, focus on including foods like carrots, sweet potatoes, spinach, kale, and liver. Yes, I did say liver. It can be tasty when prepared properly, I promise! These foods are all rich in Vitamin A and help to maintain the body's natural defenses.

Vitamin C: The Ultimate Immune Booster

Role in Immunity

VITAMIN C IS FAMOUS for its role in supporting immune health. It acts as a powerful antioxidant, protecting cells from damage caused by free radicals—unstable molecules that can harm immune function. Additionally, Vitamin C boosts the production and effectiveness of white blood cells, which are critical in the body's fight against infections.

Great Sources

THE BEST WAY TO GET Vitamin C is through foods like citrus fruits (oranges, lemons, grapefruit, etc.), strawberries, bell peppers, broccoli, and Brussels sprouts. Adding any of these into daily meals will not only boost your immune system but also improve your overall health.

Vitamin D: The Immune Regulator

Role in Immunity

VITAMIN D PLAYS A REGULATORY role in the immune system, helping it identify and respond to infections more effectively. It enhances the germ-fighting abilities of key immune cells such as monocytes and macrophages, which act as the body's infection fighters. Vitamin D also helps reduce inflammation, an important factor in maintaining overall health. Did you know that most chronic illnesses have inflammation in common? Inflammation is often at the root of the problem! More on this in a little while...

Great Sources

While sunlight is the most natural source of Vitamin D, and we typically don't get enough of it, it's important to supplement it with foods like fatty fish (salmon, mackerel), egg yolks, and (if you really must) fortified dairy products. In seasons or areas where sun exposure is limited, paying attention to these dietary sources becomes even more critical.

Vitamin E: Protection for Immune Cells

Role in Immunity

VITAMIN E IS ANOTHER potent antioxidant that plays a critical role in immune function. It helps protect immune cells from oxidative stress, which can weaken their ability to respond to infections. Vitamin E also boosts the activity of T-cells, which are vital for adaptive immunity, meaning they help your body remember and respond to specific germs. In a nutshell (see what I did there?) Vitamin E helps your body to learn - and remember - what bacteria attacked it last time and how to fight it off the next time.

Great Sources

FOODS LIKE NUTS (ALMONDS, hazelnuts), seeds, spinach, and broccoli are excellent sources of Vitamin E. Including any of these into your meals is a simple way to provide ongoing support to your immune system.

Zinc: Essential for Immune Cell Function

Role in Immunity

ZINC IS ESSENTIAL FOR the development and function of immune cells. It supports DNA synthesis, cell division, and protein production—all of which are key processes for immune health. Zinc also plays a role in wound healing and helps the body respond to inflammation and infections. It's a real fighter!

Great Sources

YOU CAN FIND ZINC IN a variety of foods, including meat, shellfish, legumes (like lentils and chickpeas), seeds, and nuts. Adding these foods to your family's diet ensures everyone gets the zinc they need to maintain a strong immune response.

Selenium: The Immune System's Antioxidant Ally

Role in Immunity

SELENIUM IS A POWERFUL antioxidant that helps protect the body from cellular damage caused by free radicals. It also supports the production of cytokines, which are molecules that help to coordinate the immune response to infections. Selenium is particularly important for enhancing the function of T-cells, which play a key role in adaptive immunity. Remember that this is the immunity you build over time. It is fuel for the system that keeps you healthy without you even realizing something was trying to make you sick in the first place!

Great Sources

TO GET ENOUGH SELENIUM, incorporate foods like Brazil nuts, seafood, meat, and eggs into your diet. These foods are not only rich in selenium but also provide a range of other essential nutrients that support overall health.

Why Whole Foods Beet (okay, "Beat") Supplements

While supplements may seem like an easy fix, they often fall short when compared to the benefits of getting your vitamins and minerals from whole foods. One reason is that supplements are not tightly regulated, meaning you might not always get what's on the label. In fact, you are more likely to get chalk than a type of calcium your body recognizes and can use! What's more, vitamins and minerals in supplements are often less bioavailable even when they are closer to the real deal, meaning your body doesn't absorb or use them as efficiently as it would from food.

For example, have you ever noticed that some supplements provide thousands of percent of your daily recommended value of a vitamin? That's because your body can only absorb a small fraction of the synthetic form found in supplements. Whole foods, on the other hand, provide these nutrients in the most natural, bioavailable form—making them easier for your body to use.

Additionally, whole foods come packed with other beneficial compounds, such as fiber, phytonutrients, and antioxidants, that supplements simply can't replicate. We don't even know what else is in the natural food, so you can bet that's missing from supplements too. By focusing on nutrient-dense foods, you're not only supporting your immune system but also benefiting your overall health in ways that supplements simply can't match.

A Natural Path to Immune Health

BUILDING A STRONG IMMUNE system is a family affair, and it starts with making smart, whole food choices. By incorporating a variety of nutrient-dense foods, you can provide your family with the vitamins and minerals needed to support their immune health. These simple, practical steps will help everyone stay healthy and resilient, season after season. So, skip the supplements whenever possible, and opt for the rich, varied nutrition that comes from real, whole foods. Your body—and your immune system—will thank you.

Antioxidants, Probiotics, and Gut Health—The Power Trio for Immune Resilience

YOUR IMMUNE SYSTEM doesn't operate in isolation; it's influenced by many factors, including the health of your cells, the balance of your gut bacteria, and the foods you eat every day. Antioxidants, probiotics, and gut health play critical roles in strengthening your body's defenses and reducing the risks of chronic illnesses. These three areas are essential for building a strong, effective immune system that can protect you from both everyday infections and long-term health challenges.

In this section, we'll explore how antioxidants from fruits and vegetables protect your immune cells, why a healthy gut microbiome is crucial for immune function, and how probiotics can enhance this vital connection. Understanding these relationships helps you make informed choices for supporting immune health naturally—for you and your entire family.

Benefits of Antioxidants from Fruits and Vegetables

Antioxidants and Their Role in Immunity

ANTIOXIDANTS ARE COMPOUNDS that help protect your body from oxidative stress, a process that can damage cells and weaken your immune system. Free radicals—unstable molecules that are produced in the body from various environmental exposures like pollution, stress, and even some foods—cause this stress. When the balance between free radicals and antioxidants tips too far in favor of free radicals, it can lead to cellular damage, inflammation, and ultimately, disease.

Free Radical Take-Down

ONE OF THE PRIMARY functions of antioxidants is to neutralize free radicals before they can cause harm. By removing these damaging molecules, antioxidants prevent them from disrupting the immune system, allowing your body to function at its peak. Sounds like a good deal to me!

Cellular Health

AS THEY PROTECT YOUR cells from oxidative damage, antioxidants are necessary to maintain the health and functionality of immune cells. This keeps your immune system running smoothly and reduces the risk of illness.

Inflammation Reduction

CHRONIC INFLAMMATION is a major contributor to weakened immune function and long-term health issues. Many antioxidants have powerful anti-inflammatory properties, which help to reduce chronic inflammation in the body. This is a big deal because approximately 125 million Americans suffer from systemic inflammation—a major factor in almost every chronic disease. In fact, chronic diseases affect more than 40% of the U.S. population and are the leading cause of death worldwide, accounting for over 50% of all deaths.

Great Sources of Antioxidants

INCORPORATING ANTIOXIDANT-rich fruits and vegetables into your daily diet is one of the simplest ways to boost immune health. Look to:

Fruits: Berries (blueberries, strawberries, raspberries), oranges, grapes, and apples.

Vegetables: Leafy greens like spinach and kale, along with bell peppers, carrots, and tomatoes.

Other (fun) sources: Green tea, dark chocolate, and nuts also provide a delicious way to add more antioxidants to your diet.

The Role of Probiotics and Gut Health in Immunity

Probiotics: Your Gut's Best Friend

PROBIOTICS ARE LIVE bacteria that are good for your gut health and, by extension, your immune system. These beneficial bacteria help maintain a balanced gut microbiome, which is essential for overall health. It's important to note that if you suspect you have small intestinal bacterial overgrowth (SIBO), consult with your doctor before starting probiotics, as they can make the condition worse - or at least increase the unpleasant symptoms. It is always a good idea to be cautious when you have gut issues. Check in with your doctor to eliminate (!) any problem diagnoses before you look at specifically increasing your intake of probiotics.

Immune Function

PROBIOTICS HELP STRENGTHEN the gut's barrier function, which prevents harmful germs from entering your bloodstream. They also help regulate the immune system by promoting the production of anti-inflammatory molecules known as cytokines and enhancing the activity of phagocytes—cells that engulf and destroy harmful invaders.

Great Sources of Probiotics

ADDING PROBIOTICS TO your diet doesn't have to be complicated. Look for sugar-free and sweetener-free options like:

- Yogurt
- Kefir
- Sauerkraut
- Kimchi
- Other fermented foods

Gut Health: The Foundation of Immune Function

Gut-Immune Connection

THE GUT IS HOME TO a significant portion of your immune system, making gut health critical to immune function. A healthy gut microbiome—a diverse population of beneficial bacteria—is essential for the development and activity of immune cells. When your gut isn't healthy, your immune system is compromised, leading to increased susceptibility to illness.

Microbiome Balance

A WELL-BALANCED GUT microbiome prevents the overgrowth of harmful bacteria and helps produce essential nutrients like B vitamins (B12, B6, Folate, etc.), which are vital for immune health. Keeping your gut balanced ensures that your immune system can respond effectively to pathogens (germs) and maintain homeostasis—keeping things in healthy equilibrium.

Immune Balance

YOUR GUT MICROBIOTA communicates with immune cells to regulate the body's response to infections and help maintain immune balance. When the gut is in balance, the immune system is better able to protect you from illness while avoiding overreactions, such as excessive inflammation.

Maintaining Gut Health

Diet

TO SUPPORT A HEALTHY gut microbiome, focus on a diet rich in fiber, fruits, vegetables, and fermented foods. These foods promote the growth of beneficial bacteria and improve gut health.

Prebiotics

PREBIOTICS ARE FIBERS that feed the good bacteria in your gut, helping them thrive. Foods like garlic, onions, asparagus, and bananas are excellent sources of prebiotics and can support a balanced microbiome.

Avoiding Antibiotic Misuse (HUGELY important!!)

THE OVERUSE OF ANTIBIOTICS is one of the most significant threats to gut health and immune function. Antibiotics don't just kill harmful bacteria; they also wipe out beneficial bacteria, disrupting the delicate balance of your microbiome. This can lead to weakened immunity and other health issues. Diarrhea and yeast infections are two of the most common health problems that stem from antibiotic use.

Please remember that antibiotics cannot treat viral infections. Taking them unnecessarily or not completing a prescribed course can harm your gut and contribute to antibiotic resistance. When you stop antibiotics early, any surviving bacteria may multiply and become resistant to that antibiotic over time. This doesn't just affect you—it affects everyone. Antibiotic resistance is becoming more common, and it means doctors must use more potent medications, often with greater risks, to treat infections that were once easily managed.

When I first became a registered nurse, MRSA (antibiotic resistant infection that can kill you) did not exist. We simply did not have this infection in hospitals! It developed over time due to the increase in use - and misuse - of antibiotics.

Strengthen Your Immune System Naturally

BY REGULARLY EATING antioxidant-rich foods, maintaining a balanced gut, and being mindful of probiotic intake, you can build a strong, resilient immune system. These natural approaches, rooted in whole foods and healthy lifestyle choices, provide your body with the tools it needs to fight off infections and reduce the risk of chronic illness. Supporting your immune health through these means isn't just for you—it benefits the entire family, helping everyone to lead healthier, more energetic and fulfilling lives.

Hydration—A Key Player in Immune Health

Water is often taken for granted or even overlooked, but it's one of the most powerful and essential elements for maintaining your body's health—including your immune system. Proper hydration ensures that every part of your body, from your cells to your brain, can function optimally. In this section, we'll explore why staying hydrated is crucial for immunity, how dehydration can hinder your body's defenses, and some simple strategies for keeping hydrated.

Understanding the importance of water (NOT sodas) and making conscious choices to stay properly hydrated will help you and your family maintain strong, responsive immune systems year-round.

Importance of Hydration and Immune Function

WATER'S ROLE IN CELLULAR Function and Detoxification

Water is a cornerstone for all cellular activities in the body, playing a direct role in how your immune system operates. Every cell in your body depends on water for transporting nutrients and flushing out waste. When you're well-hydrated, immune cells can efficiently carry out their critical functions, such as identifying and destroying harmful pathogens.

Cellular Function

In addition to aiding nutrient transport, water ensures that immune cells can communicate effectively and perform their protective roles.

Without proper hydration, this system falters, and your body becomes more vulnerable to illness.

Detoxification

Hydration also supports detoxification processes. Water helps flush toxins out of your body through urine and sweat, reducing the burden on your liver and kidneys. When these organs are functioning efficiently, the immune system can focus on fighting infections instead of dealing with excess toxins. Water also helps your gut keep things moving, preventing buildup and discomfort that can slow down immune response.

How Dehydration Can Impair Immune Response

Reduced Lymphatic Function

THE LYMPHATIC SYSTEM, which is responsible for transporting immune cells throughout the body, relies on adequate hydration to function smoothly. When you're dehydrated, this system can slow down, preventing immune cells from reaching areas where they're needed. This can reduce the efficiency of your immune response, making it harder for your body to fend off infections.

You might not be aware of these effects at first, but when you start having colds and flu more often than not, this may be the first and easiest thing to consider fixing.

Decreased Mucosal Barrier

YOUR MUCOUS MEMBRANES—LINING the respiratory and gastrointestinal tracts—are a key first line of defense against pathogens like viruses and bacteria. These membranes need adequate moisture to stay healthy and effective. Dehydration can dry them out, leaving you more susceptible to infections. Dry mucous membranes are not only less effective in blocking pathogens, but they can also become irritated and inflamed, further compromising your immune defenses.

Impaired Cellular Communication

PROPER COMMUNICATION between immune cells is critical for coordinating an effective response to invading pathogens. Dehydration can disrupt this communication, weakening your immune system's ability to respond to threats quickly and effectively.

Not only do you feel tired and sluggish when dehydrated, so does your immune defense force!

Tips for Staying Hydrated

Drink Regularly

ONE OF THE EASIEST ways to maintain proper hydration is to drink water consistently throughout the day. Don't wait until you feel thirsty—that's a sign that dehydration has already begun. A general guideline is to aim for at least 8 glasses (64 ounces, or about 2 liters) of water daily. However, your individual needs may vary based on factors such as your size, activity level, and the climate you live in. If you're larger, use larger glasses; if you're smaller, smaller glasses might work better for you.

Note: Don't chug water. Sip it so your body has time and opportunity to actually use it. If you drink too quickly, it will simply pass right through and you'll be left wondering why you are still thirsty!

Second note: You might like to add a crystal or two of Himalayan salt to a glass of water now and then during the day. This helps to keep your electrolytes in balance and can help regulate a loose digestive system.

Hydrating Foods

IN ADDITION TO DRINKING water, you can boost your hydration by incorporating water-rich foods into your diet. Cucumbers, watermelon, oranges, and strawberries are excellent options. These foods not only provide hydration but also offer valuable nutrients that support your immune system.

Monitor Urine Color

A QUICK AND EASY WAY to gauge your hydration status is by checking the color of your urine. Light yellow typically indicates you're well-hydrated, while darker yellow or amber suggests you need more fluids. Keep in mind that certain vitamins such as a B vitamin supplement and foods can alter urine color, so use this as a guideline rather than a strict rule.

Limit Dehydrating Beverages

CAFFEINATED DRINKS and alcohol can dehydrate you, so it's important to either reduce your intake or balance them out with additional water. If you do indulge, aim to drink an equal amount of water (a 1:1 ratio) to counteract the dehydrating effects.

Be Aware of Overhydration

WHILE STAYING HYDRATED is essential, it's also important not to overdo it. Drinking excessive amounts of water can flush vital vitamins, minerals, and electrolytes from your body, leading to an imbalance. Many sports drinks claim to replace these lost nutrients, but be very cautious—these drinks often contain high levels of sodium, food dyes, and sugars and/or artificial sweeteners. These ingredients come with their own health risks and cannot be considered the best solution for everyday hydration needs.

My personal choice - I would not drink the chemical concoctions.

Hydration for Optimal Immune Health

HYDRATION IS AN OFTEN-overlooked yet critical component of maintaining a healthy immune system. By ensuring that you and your family stay properly hydrated, you support the body's natural defense mechanisms—enhancing everything from cellular communication to detoxification. With a few simple habits like drinking water regularly, incorporating hydrating foods, and being mindful of what beverages you consume, you can keep your immune system strong and ready to fight off whatever comes its way.

The Critical Role of Sleep in Immune Health

Sleep is far more than a simple act of rest—it's an essential process for your overall well-being, especially when it comes to immune function. A good night's sleep gives your body time to recover, recharge, and regulate various systems that keep you healthy, including your immune defenses. In this section, we'll look at the profound link between sleep and immunity, the risks of sleep deprivation, and practical ways to improve your sleep quality.

Taking steps to prioritize sleep can strengthen your immune system and promote better health for you and your family.

The Importance of Sleep and Recovery

The Link Between Sleep and Immune Function

SLEEP IS ONE OF THE body's most effective tools for regulating and enhancing the immune system. When you sleep, your body ramps up the production of proteins called cytokines, which play a key role in targeting infections and managing inflammation. These protective proteins are particularly important when you're under stress or fighting off an illness. Without enough sleep, the production of these crucial cytokines decreases, weakening your immune defenses. So, it's no coincidence that you tend to sleep more when you're sick—your body needs that extra rest to help you heal.

Memory Consolidation for Immune Health

JUST AS YOUR BRAIN consolidates memories during sleep, your immune system does something similar. Sleep enables the immune system to "remember" the pathogens it has encountered, helping it build adaptive immunity. This means that after you've fought off an infection, your body is better prepared to respond the next time it comes across the same pathogen.

Hormonal Balance

SLEEP ALSO HELPS MAINTAIN the balance of hormones that affect your immune system, such as cortisol. Cortisol levels naturally fluctuate throughout the day, but when you're sleep-deprived, they can remain elevated, which suppresses immune function. Keeping cortisol in check through proper sleep is crucial for keeping your immune system responsive and resilient.

Effects of Sleep Deprivation on Immune Response

Increased Infection Risk

WHEN YOU DON'T GET enough sleep, your immune system takes a hit, increasing your susceptibility to infections. Research shows that people who are chronically sleep-deprived are far more likely to get sick when exposed to viruses like the common cold. Inadequate sleep weakens your immune defenses, leaving you more vulnerable to whatever is going around.

Delayed Recovery

LACK OF SLEEP DOESN'T just increase your risk of getting sick—it also slows down your recovery. When you're sleep-deprived, your body's ability to produce antibodies and mount other immune responses is compromised, which means it takes longer to fight off infections. Getting plenty of sleep while you're ill can significantly speed up your recovery.

Inflammation

AS MENTIONED EARLIER, insufficient sleep is linked to chronic inflammation. This type of persistent inflammation can contribute to a range of serious health conditions, including autoimmune disorders, cardiovascular disease, and metabolic issues. Sleep plays a vital role in keeping inflammation in check, protecting your long-term health.

Tips for Improving Sleep Hygiene

Consistent Sleep Schedule

A REGULAR SLEEP SCHEDULE is one of the most effective ways to improve your sleep quality and support your immune system. Aim to go to bed and wake up at the same time every day, even on weekends. While the occasional sleep-in won't harm you, constantly shifting your schedule can disrupt your body's internal clock, making it harder to get the restorative sleep your immune system needs.

Optimize Your Sleep Environment

CREATING A SLEEP-FRIENDLY environment is key to ensuring you get the rest your body needs. Keep your bedroom cool, dark, and quiet. If outside noise or light disturbs your sleep, consider using earplugs, an eye mask, or a white noise machine to create a more restful atmosphere.

Establish a Calming Pre-Sleep Routine

YOUR BODY NEEDS TIME to transition from wakefulness to sleep, so establish a routine that helps you wind down. Whether it's reading a book, journaling, taking a warm bath, or practicing relaxation exercises, a calming activity before bed can signal to your body that it's time to sleep.

Limit Screen Time

AVOID SCREENS—WHETHER it's your phone, tablet, or TV—at least an hour before bed. The blue light emitted from these devices interferes with the production of melatonin, the hormone responsible for regulating sleep. Reducing screen time before bed can help your body naturally prepare for rest.

Watch Your Diet

BE MINDFUL OF WHAT you consume in the hours leading up to bedtime. Large meals, caffeine, and alcohol can all disrupt your sleep. Ideally, aim to finish eating at least three hours before going to bed. Your body needs to choose between digestion and rest—and digestion will likely win out, leaving you unable to fully relax and rejuvenate.

Conclusion: Prioritize Sleep for a Strong Immune System

SLEEP IS ONE OF THE most powerful tools for maintaining and strengthening your immune system. By making sleep a priority, you give your body the time and space it needs to recover, balance hormone levels, and regulate immune responses. Simple adjustments like sticking to a consistent schedule, creating a sleep-friendly environment, and improving your pre-sleep routine can go a long way toward helping you and your family stay healthy and resilient.

There will be more on this topic later, when we look at brain health and how building good habits makes all the difference.

Building the Foundations of Immune Health

Supporting your immune system isn't just about the occasional vitamin C boost or a good night's sleep—it's a holistic, daily effort. The key is building strong foundations of immune support, starting with stress management and physical activity. When you manage stress effectively and stay active, your body is better equipped to ward off infections and maintain overall well-being. In this section, we'll dive into the connection between stress and immunity, the benefits of physical activity, and how these practices work together to strengthen your body's natural defenses.

Stress Management: Calming the Body to Strengthen Immunity

The Impact of Chronic Stress on Immunity

CHRONIC STRESS DOESN'T just make you feel overwhelmed—it can wreak havoc on your immune system. Prolonged stress triggers the constant release of cortisol, the hormone responsible for the "fight or flight" response. While this hormone is helpful in short bursts, long-term stress keeps it elevated, leading to immune suppression, weight gain and can even play a part in the development of Diabetes type 2. High cortisol levels can reduce your body's lymphocyte count, weakening your immune defenses and making you more vulnerable to infections. In essence, your body is so busy dealing with stress that it can't focus on protecting you from germs.

Inflammation: Stress's Silent Saboteur

STRESS ALSO FUELS INFLAMMATION, which, when persistent, throws your immune system out of balance. Chronic inflammation is linked to numerous health problems, including autoimmune diseases and increased susceptibility to infections. Over time, it can even contribute to more severe conditions like heart disease and cancer. When stress becomes a constant part of life, it's like a slow burn that weakens your body's defenses.

The problems brought about by chronic inflammation really can't be emphasized enough!

Behavioral Fallout from Stress

STRESS OFTEN LEADS to unhealthy lifestyle choices that further weaken the immune system. When you're stressed, you may reach for comfort foods high in sugar and fat, skip your workout, or struggle to get enough sleep. These behaviors, compounded over time, dramatically reduce your body's ability to fend off illness.

Stress Reduction Techniques: A Path to Stronger Immunity

Mindfulness

PRACTICING MINDFULNESS is one of the best ways to combat stress and lower cortisol levels. Mindful breathing, body scan meditations, and even mindful eating can help you stay present, reducing anxiety and calming the mind. By regularly practicing mindfulness, you can naturally boost your immune system's activity, making it easier for your body to defend itself.

I have included an example of a mindful eating practice for you to try, and it's available towards the end of this section.

Meditation

REGULAR MEDITATION has been shown to reduce stress hormone levels and create a sense of inner calm. It doesn't require hours of practice—even just a few minutes a day can make a significant difference. Try guided visualization, meditation apps, or even simple deep breathing to help your brain rewire its response to stress.

A key piece of information about meditation that may help: In the West, we often think it's about *not having* thoughts. Well, that's not how it works. If you are alive, your mind is working. If it's working, you are having thoughts. You can't stop them! What you *can* do is let them go. Instead of thinking "Oh, I have to make a shopping list" and then thinking about all the things that need to go on that list, you simply have the thought about the shopping list and then let it go. You have noticed it, and now you don't need to 'follow' it.

Deep Breathing

BREATHING EXERCISES like diaphragmatic breathing, 4-7-8 breathing, and box breathing can work wonders in activating your body's parasympathetic nervous system, promoting relaxation. These techniques flood your brain with oxygen, creating a state of calm that helps keep stress in check.

Bringing Relaxation Practices into Your Daily Routine

Consistency is Key

To effectively reduce stress over time, consider adding relaxation techniques into your daily routine. Set aside specific times for mindfulness, meditation, or deep breathing. The more consistent you are, the stronger your stress management habits will become.

Start Small

IF YOU'RE NEW TO RELAXATION practices, start with just five minutes a day. The idea is for this to be a time of de-stress, not distress! Gradually increase the time as you become more comfortable. Even short sessions can help reduce stress and support immune health.

Create a Relaxing Environment

A PEACEFUL ENVIRONMENT enhances the effectiveness of relaxation practices. Find a quiet, comfortable space free from distractions, and turn it into your go-to spot for relaxation. Do the best you can. You don't need a special meditation cushion or a yoga studio. Aim to make it comfortable, inviting and easeful.

And now for that promised exercise in mindful eating! This is an example of something I use with clients, and they find it to be very enlightening! The purpose here is for you to become more *aware* of what you are eating and how it affects you. We typically spend very little time focusing on what we eat and yet it is the most important thing you can do to help - or hinder - your health and wellbeing!

The results can be pretty surprising.

Are You Ready?

TRY THIS WHEN YOU ARE about to eat a meal or a snack. You'll need a journal to write in, or a paper and pen. Don't worry, it won't hurt! The best way to discover possibilities is to jump into them, so let's explore:

What do you think the food will taste like? How excited are you about it?

Write down as much as you can about why you want to eat this, and what story you are telling yourself about the reasons to eat it? (Celebration? Do you "deserve" it? Comfort?)

Bite #1 - is it as good as you thought it would be? Honestly. Is there anything about the food that is not what you expected? Write it all down!

Bite #2 - how is this bite? As good? Not so much? Keep writing!

Repeat step 2 until finished.

How was it? Did it satisfy the reason you ate it? Was it as good as you thought?

Finally, how do you feel 10, 20, 30 minutes later? How about a couple of hours later? Write it all down. Be as detailed as you can.

Repeat this process with any food you feel you can't live without. There's some deep programming going on there, so let's uncover it!

Note: Let me know how it goes!

Physical Activity and Immune Health: Move for Better Immunity

The Benefits of Moderate Movement for Immunity

Physical activity does more than keep you fit—it's a powerful way to support your immune system. Regular movement improves circulation, allowing immune cells to travel freely throughout your body. This boosts the efficiency of your immune system's surveillance abilities, helping it identify and destroy pathogens more effectively.

Reduced Inflammation

Yup. We're talking about inflammation again. Exercise promotes an anti-inflammatory environment within the body. When done in moderation, physical activity helps lower chronic inflammation, reducing the strain on your immune system and improving your overall health. "Moderation" in this case means moving often, in many different ways and not to the point of exhaustion.

You have heard of the lymphatic system by now, but did you know that it looks a lot like the circulatory system without a 'heart'? There's no pump! That's the job of regular movement - it helps the lymph to keep circulating and doing its job which is - you guessed it - keeping you healthy.

The Potential Pitfalls of Overtraining: Finding the Balance

IMMUNE SUPPRESSION from Overtraining

Yes, there can be too much of a good thing! Intense or prolonged exercise can suppress immune function, leaving you more susceptible to infections. Overtraining syndrome is marked by reaching a point of exhaustion at the end of your workout, chronic fatigue, increased illness, and longer recovery times.

Increased Risk of Illness

When you overtrain, your body becomes more vulnerable to respiratory infections and other illnesses due to elevated stress hormone levels and persistent exhaustion. Over time, this can lead to injuries and burnout.

Workout Addiction Clues

If you find it hard to take a day off from intense exercise or frequently suffer from minor, persistent injuries, it may be a sign that you're overdoing it. If your kids tell you they think you need to go to the gym on your 'rest day', it's a sign your mood may be affected. Yes, my own kids will recognise that description! Learn from my early mistakes and listen to your body. Give it the rest it needs.

Creating a Balanced Exercise Regimen

Moderate Intensity

THIS IS A CASE WHERE less is definitely more! Aim for moderate-intensity exercises, such as brisk walking, cycling, or swimming, for about 150 minutes per week. A combination of short and long workouts provides a range of benefits. The key is moderation—regular, steady movement supports immune health best. If you can walk at a good pace, and still talk, you are doing it right.

Variety is Key

MIX UP YOUR EXERCISE routine! Include a combination of aerobic activities, strength training, and flexibility exercises. It's all about balancing what you ask your body to do. Cross-training helps prevent overuse injuries and keeps your entire body in optimal shape, including your immune system. For example, if you like to go swimming, make sure you also strength train. Most importantly - make it FUN!

Rest and Recovery

ADEQUATE REST IS JUST as important as exercise. It's where the magic happens. Give your body time to recover, especially after intense workouts. Listen to your body's signals and make sure you are really balancing activity with rest.

Build Your Immune Health from the Ground Up

MANAGING STRESS AND staying active are cornerstones of immune health. By incorporating stress reduction techniques and maintaining a balanced, moderate exercise regimen, you can strengthen your immune system, reduce inflammation, and improve your overall well-being. With a few small changes, you'll be on the path to a stronger, healthier immune system for you and your family!

Advanced Strategies for Immune Support

When it comes to building a robust immune system, sometimes you need a little extra boost. While the foundation of immune health is built on everyday habits like stress management, sleep, and nutrition, there are times when turning to herbal remedies and natural supplements can give your system the extra edge it needs. In this section, we'll explore common immune-boosting herbs and supplements that can enhance your body's defenses—when used wisely and with professional guidance. Be smart and don't guess. Herbs and supplements have potent effects on the body just as much as medications do.

Herbal and Natural Supplements for Immune Health

Common Immune-Boosting Herbs

HERBS HAVE BEEN USED for centuries to strengthen the immune system, and modern science is beginning to catch up with their long-revered benefits. These herbal remedies, when taken occasionally, can help your body fight off infections and stay strong during times of stress or illness.

Don't discount or underestimate their power. Did you know that the original aspirin came from the bark of the Willow tree, for example? As wise women (and men) know, it's good stuff!

Here are some popular and effective herbs:

Echinacea

Echinacea is renowned for its ability to stimulate immune function, particularly by increasing white blood cell production. Often taken at the start of a cold, this herb can help reduce the severity and duration of cold symptoms. Its immune-enhancing properties make it a popular go-to during flu season.

Elderberry

Packed with antioxidants and vitamins, elderberry helps reduce inflammation and supports the immune system. Research has shown that elderberry can reduce the duration of flu symptoms, making it an excellent choice for boosting immune resilience during the colder months. It tastes delicious too.

Astragalus

As an adaptogen, astragalus helps your body manage stress while strengthening the immune system. It boosts white blood cell production and enhances your body's ability to fight off infections. Astragalus is particularly beneficial during periods of high stress when your immune system may need extra support.

Safe Use of Supplements: Proceed with Caution

WHILE SUPPLEMENTS ABSOLUTELY can be beneficial, it's important to approach them with care. Like exercise, supplements should be used in moderation and only after thoughtful consideration. Not all supplements are created equal—quality matters! Some brands are more reputable than others, so be sure to do your research and opt for products that are bioavailable (easily absorbed by the body).

Before adding any new supplement into your routine, it is wise to consult with your healthcare provider. They can perform the necessary tests to determine whether you truly need the supplement and, if so, how much is safe for you to take. Here are a few commonly used supplements for immune support:

Vitamin D

VITAMIN D IS ESSENTIAL for immune regulation. It helps activate immune defenses, so maintaining adequate levels is crucial, especially during the winter months when sun exposure is limited. Vitamin D can support your body's ability to fight off infections, so consider getting your levels checked to see if you need a supplement.

Note: Many people are actually deficient in Vitamin D even during summer months. There is evidence to suggest this deficiency may be caused or made worse by the liberal use of sunscreens. If this is the case for you, your provider can prescribe good quality supplements that should remedy the issue.

Zinc

ZINC PLAYS A KEY ROLE in the development and function of immune cells. However, too much zinc can actually suppress immune function, so it's important to get the dosage right. A moderate, balanced intake of zinc helps regulate immune cell production and keeps your immune response in check.

Probiotics

YOUR GUT HEALTH IS closely tied to your immune system, and probiotics can help support a healthy gut microbiome. High-quality probiotics with a variety of strains can help maintain the balance of good bacteria in your digestive system, which in turn bolsters immune function. The best quality probiotics are often found in the cooler/

refrigerator section of the health store. Long shelf life products are likely to be less effective.

Pro Tip: As mentioned earlier, the best way to get your nutrients is through whole foods. Supplements can fill occasional gaps, but eating a well-balanced diet rich in nutrients is the ideal way to support your immune health.

Consulting Healthcare Providers: Personalized Advice for Safe Supplement Use

BEFORE STARTING ANY new supplement, especially if you have underlying health conditions or are taking medications, always consult your healthcare provider. Personalized advice ensures the supplements you take are safe and tailored to your specific needs.

Your medical practitioner also needs to know about the supplements you take if you are going to take prescription medications. Some supplements can interact badly with certain medications!

Dosage and Safety

JUST BECAUSE SOMETHING is natural doesn't mean it's risk-free. The correct dosage is key to avoiding potential side effects or interactions with other medications you may be taking. Always follow professional guidance to ensure the supplements are taken in appropriate amounts and are beneficial for your health goals.

Your medical practitioner needs to know about the supplements you take if you are going to take prescription medications. Some supplements can interact badly with certain medications regardless of dosage.

By combining the wisdom of herbal remedies and supplements with professional guidance, you can safely and effectively boost your immune system when needed. But remember, the cornerstone of immune health is a balanced lifestyle—supplements are just that: a supplement, not a replacement for healthy habits.

Hygiene and Environmental Factors: Strengthening Immune Health Through Smart Habits

When it comes to safeguarding your immune system, your environment and personal hygiene play a much larger role than you might think. The good news is that there are simple, actionable steps you can take to make a real difference. From washing your hands effectively to creating a cleaner, toxin-free living space, these strategies are key to preventing illness and enhancing overall well-being. Let's dive into how you can optimize these factors to support your health.

The Importance of Hand Washing and Personal Hygiene

Preventing Infection Through Regular Hand Washing

NO, I'M NOT TAKING you back to kindergarten, but they had this right. Washing your hands with soap and water remains one of the most effective methods to prevent the spread of infectious diseases. Hand washing physically removes harmful pathogens that can cause illness, which is especially important during cold and flu seasons or when you've been in public spaces. It's simple, yet powerful.

While hand sanitizer can be a quick fix when soap and water aren't available, it's not as effective in removing certain germs, especially if your hands are visibly dirty. However, if you prefer hand sanitizer and find it convenient, it can be an additional tool in your hygiene routine. Just make sure to use one with at least 60% alcohol for maximum effectiveness.

Maintaining Strong Personal Hygiene

GOOD PERSONAL HYGIENE goes beyond just washing hands—it encompasses daily practices such as oral hygiene, regular bathing, and keeping your body clean. These habits help minimize the spread of germs and reduce the risk of infections. Think of these practices as essential layers of defense that strengthen your immune system by limiting the germs your body has to fight off.

Reducing Exposure to Environmental Toxins

Improving Indoor Air Quality

THE QUALITY OF THE air you breathe can have a direct impact on your respiratory and immune health. Good ventilation is essential, especially if you spend a lot of time indoors. Using HEPA-grade air purifiers can help eliminate indoor pollutants, allergens, and harmful particles that may compromise your immune system. Clean, fresh air is key to reducing the risk of respiratory infections.

We use HEPA-grade filters at home all year round. Five dogs and five cats produce a lot of dander and dust. It makes a big difference to the quality of the air around here! 100% recommended.

Whenever possible, open your windows to let in fresh air—provided the outdoor air quality is good and the temperature is comfortable. Not only does this keep your home well-ventilated, but it can also help you save on heating and cooling costs.

Limiting Harmful Chemicals in Your Home

BE AWARE OF THE CHEMICALS present in household cleaners, personal care products, as well as the food you eat. Many products contain toxic ingredients that can negatively affect your health over time. Opting for natural or non-toxic alternatives in your home can reduce your exposure to these harmful chemicals, ultimately supporting your immune function.

A good rule of thumb when it comes to food ingredients: If you can't pronounce it, think twice about eating it. Food labels are full of chemical additives deemed "Generally Regarded As Safe" (GRAS), but these safety standards often rely on industry-backed research. When in doubt, stick to whole, minimally processed foods to reduce your intake of unnecessary chemicals.

The same rules apply when you buy household products. Try to find natural alternatives to chemicals that require ventilation, masks and have "poison" warning labels. This stuff still gets into your body through breathing it in, via the skin on your hands etc. Yes, wearing gloves while you clean helps, but the chemicals are still there when you shower!

Feel free to reach out for simple, non-toxic recipes or suggestions on natural household alternatives!

Creating a Clean and Healthy Living Environment

Decluttering for Better Air Quality

CLUTTER CAN COLLECT dust, mold, and allergens, all of which can compromise your health, particularly if you have asthma or allergies. Keeping your living space tidy and reducing unnecessary clutter not only makes it easier to clean but also helps minimize the accumulation of these irritants. A clean, organized home is a healthier home.

Regular Cleaning for a Healthier Home

STAYING ON TOP OF A regular cleaning routine is essential to maintaining a healthy environment. Dust, mold, and other allergens can build up over time, so make sure to regularly clean your surfaces, vacuum your floors, and wash your linens. These small but consistent habits can drastically improve your indoor environment, lowering your risk of respiratory issues and allergic reactions.

Opt for Healthy, Natural Materials

CONSIDER THE MATERIALS used in your home furnishings and décor. Choosing natural options—such as wooden furniture or organic fabrics—can reduce your exposure to harmful chemicals often found in synthetic materials. Many artificial products emit volatile organic compounds (VOCs) over time, which can negatively affect air quality and health. Going natural is not only eco-friendly but also a safer option for you and your family.

By making small adjustments to your personal hygiene and home environment, you create a powerful foundation for immune health. These proactive habits will go a long way in keeping you and your family healthy year-round.

Habits vs. Willpower. Stress Reduction Habits for Better Health: Aka Your Brain and Behavior.

When it comes to creating lasting change, understanding the difference between habits and willpower is crucial. Habits, once established, run on autopilot, allowing you to perform tasks effortlessly without conscious thought. Willpower, on the other hand, is a force—an energy that, while powerful, is also finite and demanding. Think of willpower as a rocket boost—it gives you a quick surge of energy, but it's not something you can rely on long-term without burning out.

The good news is, you can make meaningful improvements in your life by creating habits that don't rely on constant supply of willpower. Here are a few strategies to help you build sustainable habits that will enhance your well-being.

Habit 1: Intermittent Fasting for Technology: Start Your Day Without Tech

Why Avoid Technology First Thing in the Morning?

TECHNOLOGY IS INHERENTLY addictive. When you wake up in the morning, your brain is especially vulnerable to influence, and reaching for your phone or laptop can set a stressful tone for the entire day. Checking emails, scrolling through social media, or glancing at your calendar can instantly overwhelm you, leading to distraction and emotional fatigue. Before you know it, you're trapped in a cycle of numbing those feelings with more mindless scrolling.

How to Break the Cycle

INSTEAD OF DIVING STRAIGHT into tech, give yourself 30-60 minutes to wake up without the screen. Use this time for other activities—meditate, journal, take a walk, or simply enjoy breakfast without the digital noise. By allowing your brain to fully wake up and engage with the day naturally, you'll find yourself more focused and productive, and your energy levels will stay balanced without relying on sheer willpower.

Habit 2. Caffeine: Friend or Foe?

Understanding Caffeine's Effects

CAFFEINE GIVES YOU a temporary energy boost by blocking adenosine, a compound that signals fatigue in the brain. While it may help you feel alert for a few hours, it doesn't address the underlying tiredness. Over time, regular caffeine consumption can lead to greater fatigue, as your body builds up adenosine while you're masking its signals. This creates a cycle where you need more caffeine to stay awake, but the crash afterward leaves you feeling drained.

Steps to Cut Back

RECOGNIZE THE IMPACT: Be mindful of how caffeine affects your body and energy levels.

Delay Your First Cup: Instead of reaching for coffee immediately, start your day with water. Hydration is key to natural energy.

Don't drink caffeine after 1pm: even if it doesn't keep you awake at night. It will still affect the *quality* of your sleep which is as important as the *quantity*.

Prioritize Sleep: Caffeine cravings are much harder to resist when you're sleep-deprived. Focus on getting enough rest so you're less tempted to rely on a morning jolt.

Take Breaks: If possible, incorporate short naps or rest periods, or go for walks during the day to replenish your energy.

By reducing your caffeine intake, you'll experience fewer energy crashes and more consistent mental clarity.

Habit 3. Pacing: A Simple Habit to Reset Your Focus

Why Pacing Works

WHEN YOU'VE BEEN WORKING for an extended period, your brain naturally seeks a break. Often, this leads to distractions like social media scrolling, which can quickly spiral into a long, unproductive session. Instead of falling into the digital black hole, try pacing. Walking around for just a few minutes allows your mind to reset without the overstimulation of negative news or endless feeds.

The Benefits of Pacing

PACING PROVIDES A SHORT mental break without dragging you into a time-consuming distraction. It gives your brain the chance to decompress, allowing your thoughts to wander freely without the need for immediate focus. Plus, it gets your blood flowing, helping to refresh both body and mind so you can return to your work with renewed energy and focus. Try it! You'll like it.

Habit 4. Give Yourself Time to Think: The Importance of Mental Downtime

IN TODAY'S FAST-PACED world, we often feel the pressure to be constantly productive. This leads to overscheduling and overstimulation, leaving little time for reflection or deep thinking. Yet, the human brain wasn't designed for non-stop activity—it needs time to process information and make thoughtful decisions.

Why We Need Downtime

WHEN WE RUSH THROUGH tasks without giving ourselves time to think, we're more likely to make hasty decisions that can lead to mistakes. Taking time to reflect not only helps you make better choices, but it also improves overall productivity in the long run. Instead of constantly reacting to stimuli, allow yourself moments of mental stillness. You'll find that your decisions become clearer and you'll spend less time correcting errors or pivoting from rushed choices.

Habit 5. Shift from Consumption to Production

The Consumption Trap

WE LIVE IN A WORLD where consuming information is easy and constant. From social media to books, podcasts, and videos, we often equate learning with progress. But endless consumption without production leaves little room for creativity and output. The more you consume, the less space you have for your own ideas to develop.

Become a Producer

TO CREATE REAL VALUE—WHETHER in writing, art, or other forms of production—you need to carve out time to engage in the creative process. And here's the key: focus on the process, not the outcome. If you set out to write a book, for example, don't let thoughts of publishing or perfectionism stop you from simply writing. Start by dedicating 10-20% of your usual consumption time to production. Whether it's journaling, brainstorming, or creating something tangible, the act of producing will shift your mindset and foster growth.

By understanding the difference between habits and willpower, you can create sustainable changes in your life that don't drain your energy. Focus on building habits that support your well-being, and reserve your willpower for when it's truly needed. Through small, intentional changes—like reducing tech use in the morning, cutting back on caffeine, and incorporating breaks—you'll improve your energy levels and mental clarity without relying on constant effort. And most importantly, by shifting from consumer to creator, you'll find yourself not just learning, but actively contributing to the world around you.

Personalized Immune Support Plan

Creating a personalized immune support plan is key to achieving lasting health and well-being. This section will guide you through the steps needed to develop a plan tailored to your individual needs and lifestyle, ensuring you can strengthen your immune system in a way that fits your daily routine.

Assessing Individual Needs and Lifestyle Factors

Personal Health Assessment

THE FIRST STEP TO BUILDING your immune support plan is to take an honest look at your current health status and lifestyle habits. Consider how your diet, exercise routine, stress levels, and sleep patterns may be impacting your immune function. Are you getting the nutrition your body needs? Is your sleep quality where it should be? Are you managing stress effectively? These questions help identify areas for improvement.

Identifying Opportunities

ONCE YOU'VE EVALUATED your current habits, the next step is to identify opportunities for positive change. Maybe your diet could use more nutrient-rich foods, or perhaps your sleep schedule needs some adjustments. Small, targeted changes in your daily routine can make a big impact on your immune health over time.

It's never too early to book your introduction call and begin your assessment!

Setting Realistic Goals and Tracking Progress

Goal Setting

SET ACHIEVABLE AND specific goals based on your assessment. For example, if you realize that you're not getting enough vitamins through your diet, you could aim to incorporate more fruits and vegetables into your meals. If stress is a major factor, you could set a goal to integrate 10 minutes of mindfulness or meditation into your daily routine. The key is to break down larger health goals into smaller, manageable steps to avoid overwhelm and build sustainable habits.

Tracking Progress

TRACKING YOUR PROGRESS is essential for seeing your progress, staying motivated and on course. You can use a journal, an app, or any method that suits your style to monitor how you're doing. Regularly review your goals and adjust them as needed, celebrating all the small wins along the way to keep the momentum going. This ongoing reflection helps ensure your plan stays effective and adaptable to your changing needs.

Adjusting the Plan for Long-Term Success

Flexibility

LIFE IS FULL OF SURPRISES, and your immune support plan should be flexible enough to adapt to those changes. As new challenges arise, whether it's a change in your work schedule, family responsibilities, or even shifts in your health, be willing to adjust your plan. What works today might need tweaking tomorrow, and that's perfectly okay. The key is to stay committed to your long-term health goals while allowing room for adjustments.

Continuous Learning

THE WORLD OF HEALTH and wellness is always evolving, and staying informed about new research and strategies for immune support is vital. Make it a habit to learn more about immune health, whether through reputable sources, new studies, or expert advice. By continuously educating yourself, you ensure that your approach remains effective and aligned with the latest evidence-based practices.

BONUS CHAPTER!
Childhood Health and Immune Wellness

Fueling Childhood Vitality Naturally

Exploration of ways to boost immune health would be incomplete without a chapter on children's health and immune wellness. Anyone who has children, or works with them, knows first-hand that when school is in session, the household is going to face round after round of respiratory infections and the like. Let's see what we can do specifically for our kids.

When it comes to keeping our children healthy, one of the most powerful tools we have is the food we give them. Proper nutrition fuels their growth, supports brain development, and perhaps most importantly, strengthens their immune system. Feeding children in a way that supports their natural vitality is not only possible—it's simpler than you might think.

In this chapter, we'll explore how to feed your child's immune system through smart, effective food choices that build lasting health. My goal is to guide you through practical strategies that don't require overhauling your life but can make a big impact on your child's well-being.

Why Nutrition Is the Foundation of a Strong Immune System

DURING CHILDHOOD, THE immune system is still developing, making kids more vulnerable to infections and illnesses. However, the right nutrition helps their bodies build resilience, fight off pathogens, and recover quickly from sickness. It's more than just protecting them from colds and flu—strong immune function also supports their overall energy, behavior, mood and even decision making skills.

What many people don't realize (unless they have read the rest of this little book) is that much of a child's immune system resides in their gut. This means that what your child eats plays a direct role in supporting healthy immune function. When you feed them with the right balance of nutrients, you're providing the building blocks they need to stay healthy, energetic, and focused.

Common Dietary Challenges in Childhood

TODAY, MANY OF THE foods marketed to children do more harm than good. From sugary cereals to ultra-processed snacks, these products may be convenient, but they don't provide the nutrients kids need. In fact, they often do the opposite, weakening their immune defenses and contributing to long-term health issues.

Here is a tip for you to explore to discover just what kind of tricks the food industry uses to con your kids into eating non-food foods.

Next time you are shopping, pick up a box of "Lucky Charms" cereal and check the list of ingredients. Not only is there a staggering amount of sugar in the list which is problematic enough, but you will also find a chemical called Trisodium Phosphate (TSP) listed. It makes the colors of the cereal brighter for longer.

Now look up your local hardware store and search for the same chemical there. You will find a box of the powder. It is used to clean the walls of your house before you paint. It is a cleaning agent to remove grease and oils from surfaces. I think if more parents knew about that, they might be less inclined to feed this to their kids. What do you think?

This is one example of cereal. It is also found in processed cheese. In fact, it can be hard to find a processed food that does NOT contain TSP or similarly unhealthy chemicals.[1]

Buyer beware!

Here are a few common dietary challenges that many parents face:

Picky (or Restrictive) Eating: It's normal for children to be selective about what they eat, but consistently avoiding nutrient-dense foods like vegetables can lead to gaps in their diet. These gaps can make it harder for their immune system to function at its best.

Excessive Sugar: Sugar is everywhere in kids' diets today, from drinks to snacks, but it has a well-documented negative effect on the immune system. Excess sugar can lead to inflammation and weaken the body's ability to fight off infections.

Processed Foods: Many processed foods are loaded with unhealthy fats, preservatives, and additives (see the example of TSP, mentioned above), which not only lack essential nutrients but also place extra strain on the body. Relying too heavily on these foods can disrupt healthy immune function over time.

How to Naturally Boost Your Child's Immune System

SUPPORTING YOUR CHILD'S immune system starts with making intentional, balanced food choices. Here are some key ways you can help your child thrive:

Prioritize Whole, Nutrient-Dense Foods

WHOLE FOODS—LIKE FRUITS, vegetables, lean proteins, and healthy fats—are packed with the vitamins and minerals that children's immune systems rely on. For instance:

Vitamin C: Found in citrus fruits, strawberries, and bell peppers, vitamin C is crucial for immune health and helps the body fend off infections.

Zinc: Foods like seeds, nuts, and legumes are excellent sources of zinc, which supports immune cell function and helps wounds heal faster.

Probiotics: Fermented foods like yogurt, kefir, and sauerkraut help build a healthy gut microbiome, which is essential for a strong immune system.

Reduce Sugar Intake

WHILE IT CAN BE DIFFICULT to avoid sugar altogether, cutting back can significantly boost your child's immune health. Sugar suppresses the immune system's ability to respond to threats, making your child more susceptible to infections. Opt for natural sweetness by incorporating fruits and other whole foods into their diet instead of sugary snacks and drinks.

Encourage a Diverse Diet

CHILDREN OFTEN GRAVITATE towards the same few foods, but encouraging variety is one of the best ways to ensure they're getting a broad range of nutrients. Aim for a colorful plate at each meal, as different colors often mean different vitamins and antioxidants. For example:

Orange and yellow foods like sweet potatoes and carrots are rich in beta-carotene, which the body converts into immune-boosting vitamin A.

Green vegetables like broccoli and spinach are packed with vitamins C and E, both critical for fighting off infections.

Limit Processed Foods

PROCESSED FOODS CAN be quick and easy, but they often contain empty calories and additives that burden the immune system. Where possible, prepare meals using whole ingredients, so you know exactly what's going into your child's body. Even small changes, like swapping out packaged snacks for fruits, veggies, or nuts, can have a big impact on their overall health.

Navigating Picky (Restrictive) Eating

PICKY EATING IS ONE of the most common challenges parents face. In fact, it may be more accurately referred to as 'restricted eating' and therein lies the true name of the problem. Restricted eating equals restricted nutrition.

It's frustrating, but understanding why it happens can help you address it more effectively. Children's taste buds are still developing, and they may be sensitive to certain flavors or textures. Repeated exposure to new foods, without pressure, can help them become more adventurous over time.

Start by offering new foods in small amounts alongside familiar favorites. Create positive associations by making meals fun and involving your child in meal prep. You don't need to turn every meal into a battle—small, consistent changes over time are the most effective.

It is not recommended to try to force the child to eat a new food. Encouragement, yes. Force, no. We all have memories of being made to eat food because of starving children in some part of the world. What that did was to a) confuse us as the food in question never actually got sent to those kids and b) we probably have a lifelong dislike of that food.

How Insight Nutrition Principles (INP) Can Help

THE INP APPROACH IS one that I created based on the science of nutrition and experience with the practicalities of working with children. I've found these principles to be incredibly effective for children as well as adults. INP focuses on whole, natural foods, free from sugar, grains, and processed ingredients. It's a simple, intuitive way of eating that helps kids develop a natural relationship with food—one that supports their immune system, energy levels, and overall well-being.

What I love about this approach is that we don't rely on rigid rules or restrictions. Instead, I encourage a shift in mindset—away from unhealthy foods and toward nutrient-rich, satisfying meals that the whole family can enjoy. When children are guided towards this way of eating, they often feel better, behave better, and develop a deeper understanding of what their bodies need to thrive.

Building a Foundation for Lifelong Health

Now that we've covered the essential building blocks of immune health, it's time to move into the practical, hands-on part of this journey. I promised at the start of this book that I wouldn't leave you with just theory. The goal was to provide actionable tools, and now you have them.

Remember, your immune system didn't get to where it is overnight, so while an immune reset may take time, the benefits can start almost immediately as you begin making small, meaningful changes. Whether it's improving your diet, prioritizing sleep, or managing stress, each step you take supports your immune health.

We'll close this section with a collection of immune-boosting recipes designed to help you and your family put the principles we've discussed into action. Full transparency: I've used AI to help generate these recipes based on the nutritional guidelines outlined in this book. Some have been tweaked by me, while others remain as they were originally generated. I'll leave it up to you to see if you can tell the difference!

Most of these recipes are vegan, making them versatile enough for almost anyone to enjoy. If you prefer, feel free to adapt them by adding your favorite proteins, or use these dishes as sides or desserts. These recipes can easily be adjusted to fit various dietary preferences—Kosher, Halal, Vegan, Vegetarian, Pescatarian—or simply be made delicious for everyone, except those following a strict carnivore plan.

I'm not advocating any specific dietary lifestyle. I've curated these recipes specifically because they incorporate the immune-boosting foods we've discussed throughout the book. These dishes are packed with essential nutrients that support your body's natural defenses and contribute to overall well-being.

And if you have children, this part is especially important: The choices you make about your child's nutrition today will have lasting effects on their health and immunity. By incorporating more whole foods, reducing sugar, and encouraging a diverse diet, you can help your child build a strong immune system that supports them through childhood and beyond. These changes don't need to be dramatic or stressful. Start small, stay consistent, and let each healthy choice build on the last. By nourishing their immune system now, you're giving your child the tools to grow into their healthiest, happiest self.

Throughout this guide, we've explored how vitamins like A, C, D, and E, along with minerals like Zinc and Selenium, are vital for immune function. Rather than relying on supplements, focus on getting these nutrients from whole foods for better bioavailability and additional health benefits.

Probiotics, hydration, and sleep are also essential to immune health, while stress management and moderate exercise are critical for reducing inflammation and boosting immune response. Herbs and natural supplements like Echinacea and Elderberry can provide an extra boost, but they should always be used under the guidance of a healthcare provider to ensure they're right for you.

Your immune health is shaped by a variety of factors, including your lifestyle, environment, and relationships. By following these recipes and incorporating the strategies in this book, you're setting yourself—and your family—up for long-lasting immune support. Remember, too, that the ingredients here are the optimal options, but if you can't find hummus without preservatives – do the best you can! Don't give up on a recipe because you can't find the exact ingredient. Eating *better* is the goal, not perfection.

Now, let's get cooking!

KIDS' DELIGHT

1. **Superhero Smoothie** *Packed with Vitamin C, antioxidants, and gut-friendly ingredients, this smoothie is a tasty way to start the day!*
    a. **Ingredients:**
        i. 1 cup spinach (rich in Vitamin A and C)
        ii. 1 ripe banana (natural sweetness and potassium)
        iii. 1/2 cup plain Greek yogurt (probiotics for gut health)
        iv. 1/2 cup mixed berries (strawberries, blueberries, or raspberries for antioxidants)
        v. 1 tablespoon chia seeds (Omega-3s for immune support)
        vi. 1/2 cup water or coconut water for hydration
    b. **Instructions:**
        i. **Place all ingredients into a blender.**
        ii. **Blend until smooth, adjusting the thickness with water or coconut water as needed.**
        iii. **Pour into a glass, and enjoy! You can even serve it with a fun straw to make it more appealing for kids.**
2. **Rainbow Veggie Wraps** (Vegan) with added options. *Kids*

love colorful foods, and these wraps are fun, crunchy, and loaded with vitamins.

　　a. **Ingredients:**
　　　　i. **1 large whole wheat or gluten-free tortilla**
　　　　ii. **1/4 cup hummus (Vitamin E for immune support)**
　　　　iii. **1/4 cup shredded carrots (Vitamin A)**
　　　　iv. **1/4 cup red bell pepper strips (Vitamin C)**
　　　　v. **1/4 cup cucumber slices (hydration and vitamins)**
　　　　vi. **1/4 cup purple cabbage, finely shredded (antioxidants)**
　　　　vii. **Optional: grilled chicken strips or turkey slices for protein**
　　b. **Instructions**:
　　　　i. Spread the hummus evenly over the tortilla.
　　　　ii. Arrange the veggies in colorful rows across the tortilla.
　　　　iii. If desired, add chicken or turkey for a protein boost.
　　　　iv. Roll the wrap tightly, slice in half, and serve!

3. **Crunchy Sweet Potato "Fries"** (Vegan) *Baked sweet potato fries are a kid-approved favorite with loads of Vitamin A and fiber.*

　　a. **Ingredients:**
　　　　i. **2 medium sweet potatoes, peeled and cut into fries**
　　　　ii. **1 tablespoon olive oil (healthy fats for immune support)**

- iii. 1/2 teaspoon garlic powder
- iv. 1/2 teaspoon paprika
- v. Salt and pepper to taste
  b. **Instructions:**
    - i. Preheat the oven to 425°F (220°C).
    - ii. Toss the sweet potato fries in olive oil, garlic powder, paprika, salt, and pepper.
    - iii. Spread the fries in a single layer on a baking sheet lined with parchment paper.
    - iv. Bake for 25-30 minutes, flipping halfway through until they're crispy on the outside and tender inside.
    - v. Serve with a side of Greek yogurt dip, flavored with a dash of lemon juice and dill.
4. **Rainbow Veggie Wraps with Hummus** (Vegan) *Packed with vitamins from colorful veggies and protein from chickpeas.*
   a. **Ingredients**:
      - i. Whole wheat or gluten-free tortillas
      - ii. 1 cup hummus (homemade or store-bought, with no added sugar or preservatives)
      - iii. 1/2 cup shredded carrots
      - iv. 1/2 cup thinly sliced red bell pepper
      - v. 1/4 cup cucumber slices
      - vi. 1/4 cup spinach leaves
      - vii. 1/4 cup purple cabbage, shredded
      - viii. 1 tbsp nutritional yeast (for a cheesy flavor and B12 boost) (see Appendix A for important information about this ingredient)
   b. **Instructions:**

i. Spread a generous layer of hummus on the tortilla.
ii. Arrange the veggies in colorful rows on top of the hummus.
iii. Sprinkle nutritional yeast over the veggies.
iv. Roll up the tortilla tightly and slice into smaller wraps for kids.
v. Serve with a side of fresh fruit like orange slices for added vitamin C.

5. **Mac & "Cheese" with Broccoli** (Vegan) *A dairy-free comfort meal that's loaded with immune-supporting garlic, turmeric, and broccoli.*
    a. Ingredients:
        i. 2 cups whole grain pasta or gluten-free pasta
        ii. 1 cup broccoli florets, steamed
        iii. 1 cup butternut squash (or sweet potato), roasted and mashed
        iv. 1/4 cup nutritional yeast (see Appendix A for important information about this ingredient)
        v. 1/2 tsp garlic powder
        vi. 1/4 tsp turmeric powder
        vii. 1 tbsp olive oil
        viii. Salt and pepper to taste
    b. Instructions:
        i. Cook the pasta according to package instructions. Drain and set aside.
        ii. In a blender, combine the roasted squash, nutritional yeast, garlic powder, turmeric, olive oil, and a splash of water

              until smooth and creamy.
- iii. Mix the sauce with the pasta and steamed broccoli.
- iv. Season with salt and pepper, then serve warm.

6. **Strawberry Banana Smoothie with Chia Seeds** (Vegan)
   This smoothie is rich in antioxidants and omega-3s for boosting immune function.

   a. **Ingredients:**
      i. 1 cup almond milk (or any plant-based milk)
      ii. 1/2 cup frozen strawberries
      iii. 1/2 banana
      iv. 1 tbsp chia seeds
      v. 1/2 tsp cinnamon (for anti-inflammatory properties)

   b. **Instructions:**
      i. Blend all ingredients until smooth.
      ii. Pour into a cup and serve with a straw or spoon for fun drinking.
      iii. Sprinkle more chia seeds on top for added texture.

7. **Berry Smoothie Bowls** - (Vegan) *This colorful smoothie bowl is easy to customize with kids' favorite toppings.*

   a. **Ingredients:**
      i. 1/2 cup frozen mixed berries (blueberries, strawberries, raspberries)
      ii. 1/2 frozen banana
      iii. 1/4 cup unsweetened almond milk
      iv. 1 tbsp chia seeds (for omega-3s)
      v. 1 tbsp almond butter
      vi. 1 tsp flaxseed meal

vii. Toppings: sliced bananas, kiwi, shredded coconut, granola

b. Instructions:
   i. In a blender, blend the frozen berries, banana, almond milk, chia seeds, almond butter, and flaxseed meal until smooth.
   ii. Pour into bowls and top with sliced bananas, kiwi, shredded coconut, and granola.
   iii. Serve immediately as a nutritious breakfast or snack!
   iv. Immune Boost: Berries are loaded with antioxidants, chia seeds and flaxseeds provide omega-3 fatty acids, and bananas add potassium for a balanced snack.

8. **Apple & Carrot Energy Bites**. (Vegan) Perfect for a quick snack or lunch box addition!
   a. Ingredients:
      i. 1 cup rolled oats
      ii. 1/2 cup grated carrot
      iii. 1/2 cup grated apple (squeeze excess juice)
      iv. 2 tbsp almond butter
      v. 1 tbsp chia seeds
      vi. 1 tbsp maple syrup
      vii. 1/2 tsp cinnamon
      viii. 1/4 tsp ground ginger
   b. Instructions:
      i. In a bowl, mix all ingredients together until well combined.
      ii. Roll the mixture into small balls (about 1 inch in diameter).

iii. Place in the fridge for 20 minutes to firm up. Store in the fridge for up to a week.
iv. Immune Boost: Apples and carrots are loaded with fiber and vitamins, chia seeds offer omega-3s, and ginger has anti-inflammatory properties.

9. **Strawberry & Citrus Salad.** (Vegan) *High in Vitamin C and Vitamin E*
    a. Ingredients:
        i. 2 cups spinach (Vitamin A and E source)
        ii. 1 cup strawberries, sliced
        iii. 1 orange, peeled and segmented
        iv. 1/4 cup almonds, sliced (Vitamin E source)
        v. 1 tbsp olive oil (Vitamin E)
        vi. 1 tbsp balsamic vinegar
        vii. Pinch of salt
    b. Instructions:
        i. In a large bowl, toss together spinach, strawberries, orange slices, and almonds.
        ii. In a small bowl, whisk together olive oil, balsamic vinegar, and salt.
        iii. Drizzle the dressing over the salad and toss gently to combine. Serve immediately.

10. **Brazil Nut Energy Balls.** (Vegan Snack) *Rich in Selenium and Vitamin E*
    a. Ingredients:
        i. 1 cup Brazil nuts (Selenium source)
        ii. 1/2 cup oats
        iii. 1/4 cup almond butter (Vitamin E source)

            iv. 1/4 cup maple syrup
            v. 1/2 cup shredded coconut
            vi. 1/2 tsp vanilla extract
            vii. Pinch of salt
    b. Instructions:
            i. In a food processor, blend Brazil nuts and oats until they form a coarse meal.
            ii. Add almond butter, maple syrup, vanilla extract, and salt. Pulse until the mixture sticks together.
            iii. Form into small balls, rolling each one in shredded coconut.
            iv. Place the energy balls in the fridge for at least 30 minutes to set before serving.
11. **Sweet Potato & Carrot Muffins.** (Vegan) *Rich in Vitamin A, Zinc, and Fiber*
    a. Ingredients:
            i. 1 cup mashed sweet potato (Vitamin A source)
            ii. 1/2 cup grated carrots (Vitamin A source)
            iii. 1/4 cup maple syrup
            iv. 1 cup oat flour
            v. 1/2 cup almond flour (Vitamin E source)
            vi. 1 tsp cinnamon
            vii. 1 tsp baking powder
            viii. 1/4 cup almond milk (or plant-based milk)
            ix. 1 tsp vanilla extract
            x. Pinch of salt
    b. Instructions:
            i. Preheat oven to 350°F (175°C).

    ii. Line a muffin tin with paper liners.
    iii. In a bowl, combine sweet potato, carrots, maple syrup, almond milk, and vanilla extract.
    iv. In a separate bowl, mix oat flour, almond flour, cinnamon, baking powder, and salt.
    v. Add dry ingredients to the wet ingredients, stirring until combined.
    vi. Scoop the batter into the muffin tin and bake for 20-25 minutes, or until a toothpick inserted comes out clean.
12. **Roasted Sweet Potato & Carrot Hummus.** (Vegan) *Rich in Vitamin A and Zinc*
    a. Ingredients:
        i. 1 medium sweet potato, roasted (Vitamin A source)
        ii. 1 large carrot, roasted (Vitamin A source)
        iii. 1 can (15 oz) chickpeas, drained and rinsed (Zinc source)
        iv. 2 tbsp tahini (Zinc source)
        v. 2 tbsp olive oil (Vitamin E source)
        vi. 1 clove garlic, minced
        vii. 1 tbsp lemon juice (Vitamin C source)
        viii. 1/2 tsp cumin
        ix. Salt and pepper to taste
    b. Instructions:
        i. Roast the sweet potato and carrot at 400°F (200°C) until tender (about 25-30 minutes).
        ii. In a food processor, combine roasted sweet

potato, carrot, chickpeas, tahini, garlic, lemon juice, cumin, and olive oil. Blend until smooth.
            iii. Add salt and pepper to taste. Serve with veggie sticks or pita for a healthy snack or appetizer.
13. **Carrot Cake Overnight Oats.** (Vegan) *Rich in Vitamin A, Fiber, and Antioxidants*
    a. **Ingredients:**
        i. 1/2 cup rolled oats
        ii. 1/4 cup grated carrot (Vitamin A source)
        iii. 1/2 cup almond milk (or plant-based milk)
        iv. 1 tbsp chia seeds (Fiber and Omega-3s)
        v. 1 tbsp maple syrup
        vi. 1/2 tsp cinnamon
        vii. 1/4 tsp nutmeg
        viii. 1 tbsp raisins (always optional)
        ix. Chopped walnuts or almonds (optional topping, Vitamin E source)
    b. **Instructions**:
        i. In a jar or bowl, combine oats, grated carrot, almond milk, chia seeds, maple syrup, cinnamon, nutmeg, and raisins.
        ii. Stir well, cover, and refrigerate overnight.
        iii. In the morning, top with chopped walnuts or almonds before serving.

COOKING FOR THE ADULT PALATE

1. **Turmeric Ginger Soup with Lentils** (Vegan) *This soothing, warming soup is filled with the anti-inflammatory ingredients turmeric and ginger, plus fiber-rich lentils for digestive and*

immune support.

a. **Ingredients:**
    i. 1 tablespoon olive oil
    ii. 1 onion, diced
    iii. 2 garlic cloves, minced (immune-boosting properties)
    iv. 1 tablespoon fresh ginger, grated (anti-inflammatory)
    v. 1 teaspoon ground turmeric (anti-inflammatory)
    vi. 1 cup red lentils (fiber and protein)
    vii. 1 can (14 oz) coconut milk (healthy fats)
    viii. 4 cups vegetable broth
    ix. 1 cup diced carrots (Vitamin A)
    x. 2 cups spinach (Vitamin C and antioxidants)
    xi. Salt and pepper to taste
    xii. Optional: A squeeze of fresh lemon juice for an added Vitamin C boost

b. **Instructions:**
    i. Heat olive oil in a large pot over medium heat. Add onion and sauté until softened, about 5 minutes.
    ii. Stir in garlic, ginger, and turmeric, cooking for another 1-2 minutes until fragrant.
    iii. Add lentils, coconut milk, vegetable broth, and carrots. Bring to a simmer and cook for about 20-25 minutes until the lentils are tender.
    iv. Stir in spinach and cook for another 2 minutes until wilted.
    v. Season with salt, pepper, and lemon juice if

using. Serve hot.
2. **Zesty Salmon with Citrus and Herb Salad** *Salmon is rich in Omega-3s, while the citrus provides a healthy dose of Vitamin C. This meal is light but full of immune-supporting ingredients.*
   a. Ingredients:
      i. 2 salmon filets (rich in Omega-3s)
      ii. 1 tablespoon olive oil
      iii. 1 garlic clove, minced
      iv. Salt and pepper to taste
      v. 2 oranges, peeled and segmented (Vitamin C)
      vi. 1 grapefruit, peeled and segmented (Vitamin C)
      vii. 2 cups mixed greens (Vitamin A and C)
      viii. 1/4 cup chopped parsley (antioxidants)
      ix. 1 tablespoon apple cider vinegar
      x. 1 tablespoon honey (natural antimicrobial properties)
   b. Instructions:
      i. **Preheat the oven to 400°F (200°C). Rub the salmon filets with olive oil, garlic, salt, and pepper.**
      ii. **Place on a baking sheet and bake for 12-15 minutes, until cooked through and flaky.**
      iii. **While the salmon bakes, prepare the salad. In a large bowl, combine orange and grapefruit segments with mixed greens and parsley.**
      iv. **In a small bowl, whisk together apple cider vinegar and honey to create the dressing.**

   v. Serve the baked salmon over the salad and drizzle with the dressing.
3. **Garlic and Lemon Sautéed Greens** (Vegan) *This quick and simple side dish pairs well with any main meal, delivering a powerful punch of immune-supporting vitamins and antioxidants.*
 a. **Ingredients:**
  i. 1 tablespoon olive oil
  ii. 2 garlic cloves, sliced thin (antiviral and antibacterial properties)
  iii. 4 cups kale or Swiss chard, stems removed and chopped (Vitamin A, C, and antioxidants)
  iv. Juice of 1 lemon (Vitamin C)
  v. Salt and pepper to taste
  vi. Optional: Red pepper flakes for a little heat
 b. **Instructions:**
  i. Heat olive oil in a large pan over medium heat.
  ii. Add garlic slices and sauté for 1-2 minutes until fragrant, being careful not to burn them.
  iii. Add the greens and sauté for about 5 minutes, until they begin to wilt.
  iv. Squeeze lemon juice over the greens and season with salt, pepper, and red pepper flakes if using.
  v. Serve hot as a side to your favorite protein.
4. **Lentil & Sweet Potato Stew** (Vegan) *Rich in beta-carotene, fiber, and plant protein, this stew offers comforting immune support.*
 a. **Ingredients:**

         i. 1 cup dried lentils (green or brown), rinsed
         ii. 1 medium sweet potato, peeled and diced
         iii. 1 small onion, chopped
         iv. 2 garlic cloves, minced
         v. 1-inch piece of fresh ginger, grated
         vi. 1 tsp turmeric
         vii. 1 tsp cumin
         viii. 1/2 tsp smoked paprika
         ix. 4 cups vegetable broth
         x. 2 cups spinach or kale, roughly chopped
         xi. Salt and pepper to taste
    b. Instructions:
         i. In a large pot, sauté the onion, garlic, and ginger until fragrant.
         ii. Add the turmeric, cumin, and paprika and cook for another minute.
         iii. Add the sweet potato, lentils, and vegetable broth. Bring to a boil.
         iv. Reduce heat and simmer for 20-25 minutes, until lentils and sweet potatoes are tender.
         v. Stir in the spinach or kale, and cook for another 5 minutes.
         vi. Season with salt and pepper, and serve hot with a slice of whole-grain bread.
5. **Immune-Boosting Green Power Bowl** (Vegan) *Loaded with antioxidant-rich greens, healthy fats, and protein.*
    a. Ingredients:
         i. 1/2 cup cooked quinoa
         ii. 1/4 cup chickpeas, roasted or steamed
         iii. 1/4 avocado, sliced

iv. 1 cup mixed greens (spinach, kale, arugula)
v. 1/4 cup shredded carrots
vi. 1 tbsp pumpkin seeds (rich in zinc)
vii. 1 tbsp hemp seeds (rich in omega-3s)
viii. 2 tbsp tahini dressing (blend tahini, lemon juice, garlic, and water)
ix. 1/4 tsp black pepper (enhances turmeric absorption, if added)
  b. **Instructions:**
     i. In a bowl, layer the quinoa, chickpeas, and greens.
     ii. Top with avocado slices, shredded carrots, pumpkin seeds, and hemp seeds.
     iii. Drizzle with tahini dressing and sprinkle with black pepper.
     iv. Serve immediately, either warm or at room temperature.
6. **Mushroom & Miso Soup** (Vegan) *Miso and mushrooms are rich in probiotics and antioxidants, making this soup a great immune booster.*
   a. **Ingredients**:
      i. 4 cups vegetable broth
      ii. 1 cup mushrooms (shiitake or button), sliced
      iii. 2 tbsp miso paste
      iv. 1 clove garlic, minced
      v. 1-inch piece of fresh ginger, grated
      vi. 1/2 cup tofu, cubed (optional)
      vii. 2 green onions, chopped
      viii. 1 tbsp sesame oil
      ix. 1 tbsp soy sauce (or tamari for gluten-free)

                x. 1/2 cup chopped spinach or bok choy
    b. **Instructions**:
                i. In a large pot, sauté the garlic and ginger in sesame oil until fragrant.
                ii. Add the mushrooms and cook for 3-4 minutes until softened.
                iii. Pour in the vegetable broth and soy sauce, and bring to a simmer.
                iv. Stir in the miso paste until dissolved.
                v. Add tofu and spinach, cooking for another 5 minutes.
                vi. Garnish with chopped green onions and serve hot.
7. **Creamy Sweet Potato & Lentil Soup** (Vegan) A warming, creamy soup that's nutrient-dense and satisfying for colder days.
    a. **Ingredients**:
                i. 1 medium sweet potato, peeled and cubed
                ii. 1/2 cup red lentils, rinsed
                iii. 1 small onion, chopped
                iv. 2 cloves garlic, minced
                v. 1/2 tsp turmeric (anti-inflammatory)
                vi. 1/2 tsp cumin
                vii. 3 cups vegetable broth
                viii. 1 tbsp olive oil
                ix. Salt and pepper to taste
                x. Fresh cilantro for garnish
    b. **Instructions**:
                i. Heat olive oil in a pot and sauté onion and garlic until softened.
                ii. Add sweet potato, lentils, turmeric, and cumin. Stir for 1 minute.

iii. Pour in vegetable broth and bring to a boil. Lower the heat and simmer for 20 minutes, until the lentils and sweet potatoes are soft.
iv. Use an immersion blender to blend the soup to your desired creaminess.
v. Season with salt and pepper. Garnish with fresh cilantro.
vi. Immune Boost: Sweet potatoes offer vitamin A, lentils are rich in protein and zinc, and turmeric provides anti-inflammatory benefits.

8. **Quinoa Stuffed Bell Peppers** (Vegan) *Hearty and nutritious, these stuffed peppers are perfect for a light lunch or dinner.*
    a. **Ingredients:**
        i. 4 large bell peppers (red, yellow, or orange)
        ii. 1 cup cooked quinoa
        iii. 1/2 cup black beans (canned, drained, and rinsed)
        iv. 1/4 cup diced tomatoes
        v. 1 small zucchini, diced
        vi. 1/2 tsp cumin
        vii. 1/2 tsp smoked paprika
        viii. 2 tbsp nutritional yeast (for a cheesy flavor) (see Appendix A for important information about this ingredient)
        ix. Salt and pepper to taste
        x. Fresh parsley for garnish
    b. **Instructions:**
        i. Preheat the oven to 375°F (190°C). Cut the tops off the bell peppers and remove the seeds.

- ii. In a pan, sauté diced zucchini with cumin and smoked paprika. Add quinoa, black beans, and diced tomatoes. Stir until well combined.
- iii. Season with salt, pepper, and nutritional yeast.
- iv. Stuff the peppers with the quinoa mixture and place them in a baking dish.
- v. Bake for 25-30 minutes, until the peppers are tender. Garnish with fresh parsley.
- vi. Immune Boost: Quinoa is high in protein and zinc, black beans provide fiber and immune-supporting nutrients, and bell peppers are packed with vitamin C.

9. **Garlic & Lemon Zoodles** (Vegan) *Light and refreshing, this dish is ideal for a quick immune-boosting lunch.*
    a. **Ingredients**:
        i. 2 medium zucchinis, spiralized into zoodles
        ii. 2 cloves garlic, minced
        iii. 1 tbsp olive oil
        iv. Juice of 1 lemon
        v. 1/4 cup cherry tomatoes, halved
        vi. 2 tbsp hemp seeds (for extra protein and zinc)
        vii. Salt and pepper to taste
        viii. Fresh basil for garnish
    b. **Instructions**:
        i. Heat olive oil in a large pan and sauté garlic until fragrant.
        ii. Add zoodles and cherry tomatoes, and

sauté for 2-3 minutes until slightly tender.
      iii. Remove from heat, stir in lemon juice, and season with salt and pepper.
      iv. Top with hemp seeds and fresh basil. Serve immediately!
      v. Immune Boost: Garlic is a powerful immune booster, lemon provides vitamin C, and hemp seeds offer protein and essential fatty acids.

10. **Chickpea & Spinach Stir-Fry** (Vegan) *Rich in Zinc, Selenium, and Vitamin A*
    a. **Ingredients**:
        i. 1 can (15 oz) chickpeas, drained and rinsed (Zinc source)
        ii. 2 cups spinach (Vitamin A and E source)
        iii. 1 clove garlic, minced
        iv. 1 tbsp olive oil
        v. 1 tbsp lemon juice (Vitamin C source)
        vi. 1 tsp ground cumin
        vii. 1/2 tsp paprika
        viii. Salt and pepper to taste
        ix. Brazil nuts for garnish (Selenium source)
    b. **Instructions**:
        i. Heat olive oil in a large skillet over medium heat. Add garlic and cook until fragrant.
        ii. Add chickpeas, cumin, and paprika, stirring until chickpeas are heated through and slightly browned (about 5 minutes).
        iii. Toss in spinach and cook until wilted.
        iv. Drizzle with lemon juice, season with salt and pepper.
        v. Serve with chopped Brazil nuts for added

selenium.

11. **Zesty Broccoli & Almond Stir Fry** (Vegan) *Packed with Vitamin C, Vitamin E, and Zinc*
    a. **Ingredients**:
        i. 2 cups broccoli florets (Vitamin C and E source)
        ii. 1/4 cup almonds, sliced (Vitamin E source)
        iii. 1 red bell pepper, sliced (Vitamin C source)
        iv. 1 tbsp sesame seeds (Zinc source)
        v. 1 tbsp olive oil
        vi. 2 tbsp soy sauce
        vii. 1 tsp ginger, minced
        viii. 1 clove garlic, minced
        ix. 1 tsp lemon zest
        x. Salt and pepper to taste
    b. **Instructions**:
        i. Heat olive oil in a pan over medium heat. Add garlic and ginger, sauté until fragrant.
        ii. Add broccoli, red bell pepper, and a splash of water. Cook until tender, about 5 minutes.
        iii. Stir in soy sauce and lemon zest.
        iv. Add almonds and sesame seeds, stirring for an additional 2 minutes. Season with salt and pepper before serving.
12. **Kale & Quinoa Power Bowl** (Vegan)*High in Vitamin A, Zinc, and Selenium*
    a. **Ingredients**:
        i. 1 cup cooked quinoa (Zinc source)
        ii. 2 cups kale, chopped (Vitamin A source)
        iii. 1 avocado, sliced (Vitamin E source)
        iv. 1/4 cup pumpkin seeds (Zinc source)

- v. 1 tbsp olive oil (Vitamin E source)
- vi. 1 tbsp lemon juice (Vitamin C source)
- vii. Salt and pepper to taste

b. **Instructions**:
  - i. Massage kale with olive oil and lemon juice until softened.
  - ii. In a bowl, layer quinoa, kale, avocado, and pumpkin seeds.
  - iii. Season with salt and pepper and enjoy as a nutrient-packed meal.

13. **Zucchini & Almond Fritters** (Vegan) *Packed with Vitamin E, Zinc, and Fiber*
    a. Ingredients:
        - i. 2 medium zucchinis, grated
        - ii. 1/4 cup almond flour (Vitamin E source)
        - iii. 1/4 cup chickpea flour (Zinc source)
        - iv. 2 tbsp ground flaxseed mixed with 5 tbsp water (egg substitute)
        - v. 1/4 cup finely chopped onion
        - vi. 2 tbsp fresh parsley, chopped
        - vii. 1 tsp ground cumin
        - viii. 1/2 tsp paprika
        - ix. Salt and pepper to taste
        - x. Pure Olive oil for frying (Vitamin E source)
    b. **Instructions**:
        - i. Grate the zucchinis and squeeze out excess moisture with a clean towel.
        - ii. In a bowl, combine grated zucchini, almond flour, chickpea flour, onion, parsley, cumin, paprika, and the flaxseed mixture.

iii. Form the mixture into small patties.
iv. Heat olive oil in a skillet over medium heat. Fry the fritters on each side until golden brown (about 3-4 minutes per side).
v. Serve with a side of lemon-tahini sauce or a green salad.

14. **Lentil & Spinach Stew** (Vegan) *Packed with Zinc, Iron, and Vitamin A*
    a. **Ingredients**:
        i. 1 cup dried lentils (Zinc source)
        ii. 2 cups fresh spinach (Vitamin A and E source)
        iii. 1 onion, chopped
        iv. 2 cloves garlic, minced
        v. 1 can (15 oz) diced tomatoes
        vi. 1 tbsp olive oil
        vii. 1 tsp ground cumin
        viii. 1 tsp smoked paprika
        ix. 4 cups vegetable broth
        x. Salt and pepper to taste
    b. **Instructions**:
        i. Heat olive oil in a large pot over medium heat. Add onions and garlic, sauté until softened.
        ii. Add lentils, cumin, and paprika, stirring for 1-2 minutes.
        iii. Add vegetable broth and diced tomatoes, bring to a boil, then reduce heat and simmer for 25-30 minutes until lentils are tender.
        iv. Stir in spinach and cook for another 5 minutes until wilted.

v. Season with salt and pepper before serving.

15. **Sautéed Brussels Sprouts with Almonds** (Vegan) *Packed with Vitamin C, Vitamin E, and Fiber*
    a. **Ingredients**:
        i. 2 cups Brussels sprouts, halved (Vitamin C source)
        ii. 1/4 cup slivered almonds (Vitamin E source)
        iii. 1 tbsp olive oil (Vitamin E source)
        iv. 1 clove garlic, minced
        v. 1 tbsp lemon juice (Vitamin C source)
        vi. Salt and pepper to taste
    b. **Instructions**:
        i. Heat olive oil in a large skillet over medium heat. Add garlic and sauté until fragrant.
        ii. Add Brussels sprouts and cook for 8-10 minutes, stirring occasionally, until they are tender and slightly crispy.
        iii. Stir in slivered almonds and cook for an additional 2-3 minutes.
        iv. Drizzle with lemon juice and season with salt and pepper before serving.

16. **Pumpkin & Lentil Curry** (Vegan) *Rich in Vitamin A, Zinc, and Fiber*
    a. **Ingredients**:
        i. 1 cup cubed pumpkin (Vitamin A source)
        ii. 1/2 cup dried lentils (Zinc source)
        iii. 1 onion, chopped
        iv. 2 cloves garlic, minced
        v. 1 tbsp curry powder
        vi. 1/2 tsp turmeric (anti-inflammatory)
        vii. 1 can (15 oz) coconut milk

           viii. 1 cup vegetable broth
            ix. 2 tbsp fresh cilantro, chopped (optional garnish)
             x. Salt and pepper to taste
    b. **Instructions**:
             i. In a large pot, heat olive oil over medium heat. Add onions and garlic, cook until soft.
            ii. Stir in curry powder and turmeric, then add pumpkin and lentils. Cook for 2-3 minutes.
           iii. Pour in coconut milk and vegetable broth. Bring to a boil, then reduce heat and simmer for 25-30 minutes until lentils and pumpkin are tender.
            iv. Season with salt and pepper and garnish with fresh cilantro before serving.
17. **Citrus & Avocado Salad** (Vegan) *Rich in Vitamin C, Vitamin E, and Healthy Fats*
    a. **Ingredients**:
             i. 2 oranges, peeled and segmented (Vitamin C source)
            ii. 1 avocado, sliced (Vitamin E source)
           iii. 1/4 cup pomegranate seeds (Vitamin C source)
            iv. 1/4 cup slivered almonds (Vitamin E source)
             v. 1 tbsp olive oil (Vitamin E source)
            vi. 1 tbsp lemon juice
           vii. Salt and pepper to taste
    b. **Instructions**:
             i. Arrange orange segments and avocado slices on a plate.
            ii. Sprinkle with pomegranate seeds and

slivered almonds.
iii. Drizzle with olive oil and lemon juice, and season with salt and pepper before serving.

Conclusion: A New Chapter in Your Health Journey

As you've discovered throughout this book, your immune system is a powerful ally, and nourishing it naturally is key to lifelong health, wellness and quality of life. By incorporating immune-boosting foods, adopting healthier habits, and paying attention to your body's needs, you're setting yourself and your family on a path to lasting wellness. Every small change you make, from the foods you eat to the routines you follow, is a choice. What you choose to do can strengthen your resilience and give you more life in your years. Today's world needs a special approach if you are to do more than survive - thrive.

But this journey doesn't end here. If you're ready to dive deeper into personalized solutions, tailored strategies, and advanced guidance, I invite you to take the next step. Whether you're dealing with specific health concerns, looking to optimize your nutrition, or wanting to transform your relationship with food, I'm here to help.

Let's Connect

I offer one-on-one consultations and advanced nutrition coaching programs that go beyond what's covered in this book. Together, we can craft a customized plan designed to meet your unique needs, help you overcome challenges, and reach your health goals. Your immune system—and your whole body—deserves the best care possible, and I'm excited to be involved in part of that journey with you.

Contact Me Today

If you're ready to take action, reach out for a personal consultation or sign up for my advanced nutrition coaching program. Let's unlock your full potential and build a healthier, more healthy and fulfilling future.

You can reach me at https://app.paperbell.com/packages/72639, or visit my website at www.gaffenstone.com[1] to book your complimentary consultation session.

Your best health is within reach—let's get started!

MICHAELA

---

1. http://www.gaffenstone.com

Appendix A: Nutritional Yeast

A note of caution about Nutritional yeast:
Nutritional yeast is a great source of dietary fiber, but because of its high fiber content, it's a good idea to introduce it gradually into your diet. Starting slow can help prevent any potential abdominal discomfort.

For some people, nutritional yeast can trigger headaches. It contains compounds including tyramine, which can be a migraine trigger. If you sometimes experience migraines, it may be best to avoid nutritional yeast to prevent provoking this problem.

Nutritional yeast is also rich in niacin (vitamin B3). While facial flushing from niacin is usually harmless, consuming large amounts of it can lead to other, more concerning side effects. It's important to be mindful of your intake.

Some studies suggest that dietary yeast could significantly increase symptoms in certain individuals with inflammatory bowel disease (IBD). If you have IBD, consider consulting with a healthcare provider before incorporating nutritional yeast into your meals.

Lastly, but perhaps most significantly, something to be aware of - nutritional yeast grows easily and well. That means it can be grown from 'good' food and it can be grown with poor quality food. Knowing your source is very important, and I suggest you use it sparingly, just to be safe.

That said...

Benefits of Nutritional Yeast

Boosting Energy

NUTRITIONAL YEAST IS often fortified with vitamin B-12, but it's important to check the label, as not all brands include it. Vitamin B-12 can help boost energy levels, as a deficiency in this essential nutrient can lead to fatigue and weakness. This makes fortified nutritional yeast particularly valuable for vegetarians and vegans, as B-12 is primarily found in animal products. Adults need around 2.4 mcg of vitamin B-12 daily, and just a quarter-cup of fortified nutritional yeast can provide more than seven times this amount, making it an excellent source for those looking to increase their intake.

Supporting the Immune System

RESEARCH INDICATES that Saccharomyces cerevisiae, the strain of yeast found in nutritional yeast, can support immune function and reduce inflammation caused by bacterial infections. Nutritional yeast may also aid in managing diarrhea, offering an additional immune-supportive benefit.

Promoting Skin, Hair, and Nail Health

NUTRITIONAL YEAST HAS been linked to improvements in skin, hair, and nail health. Some studies suggest it may help strengthen brittle nails, reduce hair loss, and improve acne, making it particularly beneficial during adolescence when skin concerns are more common.

Improving Glucose Sensitivity

WHILE THERE IS A BELIEF that nutritional yeast may help improve glucose sensitivity in people with type 2 diabetes, further research is needed to confirm this. However, studies on chromium-enriched yeast, typically brewer's yeast, have shown potential in lowering fasting blood glucose levels and cholesterol in animal models, indicating that certain types of yeast may have positive effects on blood sugar management.

Supporting a Healthy Pregnancy

NUTRITIONAL YEAST CAN be a helpful addition to a healthy pregnancy diet. The U.S. Preventive Services Task Force recommends that women planning pregnancy take 400–800 mcg of folic acid daily to support fetal development and prevent congenital abnormalities. Since many brands of nutritional yeast are fortified with folic acid, it can be a convenient way for pregnant women to meet their folic acid needs. However, some brands may contain more than the recommended amount, so it's always a good idea to consult a healthcare provider before using it as a supplement during pregnancy.

Appendix B: Resources and further reading:

Nutrition and Immune System Function:

- **Calder, P. C. (2020). "Nutrition, Immunity, and COVID-19."** BMJ Nutrition, Prevention & Health, 3(1), 74-92.
  This paper discusses how various nutrients (such as vitamins, minerals, and fatty acids) support immune function and the potential role of nutrition in fighting infections like COVID-19.
  [Link: https://nutrition.bmj.com/][1]
- **Gombart, A. F., Pierre, A., & Maggini, S. (2020). "A Review of Micronutrients and the Immune System – Working in Harmony to Reduce the Risk of Infection."** Nutrients, 12(1), 236.
  This review examines the role of key micronutrients (like vitamin C, D, and zinc) in immune system support and disease prevention.
  [Link: https://www.mdpi.com/][2]

Gut Health and Immunity:

- **Zmora, N., Suez, J., & Elinav, E. (2018). "You Are What You Eat: Diet, Health, and the Gut Microbiota."** Nature Reviews Gastroenterology & Hepatology, 15(1), 53-64.

---

1. https://nutrition.bmj.com/%5d
2. https://www.mdpi.com/

This review explores the complex interaction between diet, gut microbiota, and immune responses, highlighting the importance of gut health in maintaining overall immunity.
[Link: https://www.nature.com/[3]]
- **Belkaid, Y., & Harrison, O. J. (2017). "Homeostatic Immunity and the Microbiota."** Immunity, 46(4), 562-576.
This paper provides insights into how the gut microbiota regulates the immune system and its importance for preventing immune-related disorders.
[Link: https://www.cell.com/immunity/][4]

Lifestyle and Immune Function:

- **Campbell, J. P., & Turner, J. E. (2018). "Debunking the Myth of Exercise-Induced Immune Suppression: Redefining the Impact of Physical Activity on Immunity."** Exercise Immunology Review, 24, 45-55.
This article offers a new perspective on how regular physical activity can enhance rather than suppress the immune system.
[Link: https://eir-isei.de/[5]]
- **Nieman, D. C. (1994). "Exercise, Infection, and Immunity."** International Journal of Sports Medicine, 15(3), S131-S141.
A foundational study on the impact of physical exercise on immune function, supporting the importance of regular movement in bolstering immunity.
[Link: https://www.thieme-connect.com/[6]]

---

3. https://www.nature.com/

4. https://www.cell.com/immunity/%5d

5. https://eir-isei.de/

6. https://www.thieme-connect.com/

Sleep and Immune Health:

- **Besedovsky, L., Lange, T., & Born, J. (2012). "Sleep and Immune Function."** Pflügers Archiv - European Journal of Physiology, 463, 121–137.
  This paper reviews the vital connection between sleep quality, sleep cycles, and immune function.
  [Link: https://link.springer.com/[7]]
- **Irwin, M. R. (2019). "Sleep and Inflammation: Partners in Sickness and in Health."** Nature Reviews Immunology, 19(11), 702-715.
  This review details how poor sleep can drive inflammation and weaken immune function, making it essential for immune health.
  [Link: https://www.nature.com/[8]]

Mind-Body Connection and Immunity:

- **Glaser, R., & Kiecolt-Glaser, J. K. (2005). "Stress-Induced Immune Dysfunction: Implications for Health."** Nature Reviews Immunology, 5(3), 243-251.
  This paper highlights how chronic stress impairs immune function and the importance of stress management for immune health.
  [Link: https://www.nature.com/[9]]
- **Dhabhar, F. S. (2014). "Effects of Stress on Immune Function: The Good, the Bad, and the Beautiful."** Immunologic Research, 58, 193–210.

---

7. https://link.springer.com/

8. https://www.nature.com/

9. https://www.nature.com/

This research delves into the different types of stress and how acute and chronic stress can impact immune responses.
[Link: https://link.springer.com/[10]]

Brain Health and Eating Behavior:

- **Gibson, E. L. (2006). "Emotional Influences on Food Choice: Sensory, Physiological and Psychological Pathways."** Physiology & Behavior, 89(1), 53-61.
This article examines how emotions affect food choices and eating behavior, focusing on the brain's reward and stress systems.
[Link: https://www.sciencedirect.com/[11]]
- **Berthoud, H. R. (2011). "Metabolic and Hedonic Drives in the Neural Control of Appetite: Who is the Boss?"** Current Opinion in Neurobiology, 21(6), 888-896.
This paper discusses how the brain's hedonic (pleasure-based) and metabolic systems interact to influence eating behavior and food cravings.
[Link: https://www.sciencedirect.com/[12]]

Emotional Eating and Brain Function:

- **Konttinen, H. (2020). "Emotional Eating and Obesity: The Role of Stress and Self-Regulation in Eating Behavior."** Current Obesity Reports, 9, 252–261.
This review explores the links between emotional eating, stress, and brain mechanisms, highlighting self-regulation

---

10. https://link.springer.com/

11. https://www.sciencedirect.com/

12. https://www.sciencedirect.com/

challenges that lead to overeating.
[Link: https://link.springer.com/[13]]
- **Adam, T. C., & Epel, E. S. (2007). "Stress, Eating, and the Reward System."** Physiology & Behavior, 91(4), 449-458.
This article discusses how stress influences eating behaviors by activating the brain's reward system, leading to emotional eating and potential weight gain.
[Link: https://www.sciencedirect.com/[14]]

Neuroscience of Emotional Eating:

- **Sinha, R., & Jastreboff, A. M. (2013). "Stress as a Common Risk Factor for Obesity and Addiction."** Biological Psychiatry, 73(9), 827-835.
This paper discusses how stress activates brain circuits involved in both emotional eating and addictive behaviors, linking obesity to emotional dysregulation.
[Link: https://www.sciencedirect.com/[15]]
- **Tomiyama, A. J. (2019). "Stress and Obesity."** Annual Review of Psychology, 70(1), 703-718.
This review focuses on the relationship between chronic stress, emotional eating, and brain function in contributing to obesity.
[Link: https://www.annualreviews.org/[16]]

---

13. https://link.springer.com/

14. https://www.sciencedirect.com/

15. https://www.sciencedirect.com/

16. https://www.annualreviews.org/

Behavioral Interventions and Emotional Eating:

- **Van Strien, T. (2018). "Causes of Emotional Eating and Matched Treatment of Obesity."** Current Diabetes Reports, 18(6), 35.
  This article outlines the psychological triggers of emotional eating and offers evidence-based behavioral strategies for managing emotional eating.
  [Link: https://link.springer.com/[17]]
- **Forman, E. M., & Butryn, M. L. (2015). "A New Look at the Science of Weight Control: How Acceptance and Commitment Strategies Can Address Emotional and Addictive Eating."** Journal of Contextual Behavioral Science, 4(3), 169-177.
  This study introduces behavioral approaches like Acceptance and Commitment Therapy (ACT) for managing emotional eating and promoting healthy eating behaviors.
  [Link: https://www.sciencedirect.com/[18]]

Gut-Brain Axis and Emotional Eating:

- **Cryan, J. F., O'Riordan, K. J., & Cowan, C. S. M. (2019). "The Microbiota-Gut-Brain Axis: From Cognition to Mental Health."** Physiological Reviews, 99(4), 1877-2013.
  This review explores how the gut microbiota interacts with the brain to influence behavior, emotions, and eating patterns, linking gut health to emotional eating.
  [Link: https://journals.physiology.org/][19]

---

17. https://link.springer.com/
18. https://www.sciencedirect.com/

- **Mayer, E. A. (2011). "Gut Feelings: The Emerging Biology of Gut-Brain Communication."** Nature Reviews Neuroscience, 12(8), 453-466.
  This paper highlights the role of the gut-brain axis in regulating emotions and how it may contribute to emotional eating patterns.
  [Link: https://www.nature.com/[20]]

Mindfulness and Emotional Eating:

- **Katterman, S. N., Kleinman, B. M., Hood, M. M., Nackers, L. M., & Corsica, J. A. (2014). "Mindfulness Meditation as an Intervention for Binge Eating, Emotional Eating, and Weight Loss: A Systematic Review."** Eating Behaviors, 15(2), 197-204.
  This review explores the effectiveness of mindfulness meditation for reducing emotional eating and promoting better self-regulation of food intake.
  [Link: https://www.sciencedirect.com/[21]]
- **Tapper, K. (2018). "Mindfulness and Weight Loss: A Systematic Review."** Obesity Reviews, 19(2), 212-223.
  This review looks at how mindfulness can be used to help manage emotional eating and support long-term weight management.
  [Link: https://onlinelibrary.wiley.com/[22]]

---

19. https://journals.physiology.org/%5d

20. https://www.nature.com/

21. https://www.sciencedirect.com/

22. https://onlinelibrary.wiley.com/

[1] For more information, see https://forum.facmedicine.com/threads/understanding-trisodium-phosphate-safety-and-health-effects.80989/